My Stroke: 450 Days From Severe Aphasia To Speaking, Reading And Writing

Donald F. Weinstein, Ph.D

This book is available through the National Aphasia Association. For details, visit   or write/call:

National Aphasia Association,
350 Seventh Avenue, Suite 902,
New York, NY 10001
(800) 922-4622

Printed in the United States of America

Library of Congress Cataloging- in –Publication Data

Weinstein, Donald F

My stroke: 450 days from severe aphasia to speaking, reading and writing by Donald F. Weinstein

Includes index

1. Stroke victim – The effects of severe aphasia.
2. Stroke survivor- The struggle to speak, read and write.
3. Caregivers and supporters – The multitude of ways they help and the stress they feel.
4. Insurance companies- Their role in speech therapy

I. Title

The author is neither a medical doctor nor a psychologist. This book can not replace the services of a qualified health professional. The author and publisher shall not be held responsible for any loss or damage allegedly arising from any information, thoughts, ideas or suggestions in this book.

ISBN- 13   978-0-615-23123-5
ISBN- 10   0-615-23123-3

For Dale, Jeff, Anne, Alison,
Jessica and Peggy

Table of Contents

Preface – My Stroke

By Risha W. Levinson, DSW
Professor Emerita
Adelphi University
School of Social Work

Aphasia is a language disorder in which there is an impairment of the ability to process language but does not affect intelligence. Depending on the area and extent of the damage, someone suffering from aphasia may be able to speak but not read or write, or vice versa, or display any of a wide variety of other deficiencies in language comprehension and production, such as being able to sing but not speak. Famous people with aphasia include Maurice Ravel, Jan Berry of the singing group Jan and Dean, Ralph Waldo Emerson, Robert E. Lee, the playwright Joseph Chaikin, and the ABC television journalist Bob Woodruff.

The prognosis of those with aphasia varies widely, and is dependent upon age of the patient, site and size of lesion, and type of aphasia. The key to improved functioning depends very much on the patient's drive, effort, and ability to persevere over frustration. This book is a testament to one such patient, Donald Weinstein, who has managed to "come back" from a severe form of this condition.

In 2002, Weinstein suffered an embolic cerebrovascular accident with severe aphasia. After being in the hospital for the critical phase of his illness he entered Transitions of Long Island, a comprehensive neuro-rehabilitation program for individuals with acquired neuralgic injuries, including traumatic brain injury, stroke, brain tumor, anoxia, encephalitis, mild head injury and other brain diseases. He couldn't speak, read, write, sing or do arithmetic. Fifteen months later he was able to read classic, write professional reports, sing at a Passover Seder, manage numerical data and, mirabile dictum, take a vacation trip to Puerto Rico.

Among the most important factors to his recovery, from the limitations of his condition, were the love and devotion of his family, the guidance and support of caring professionals, the cheering from the sidelines of special friends, and above all his determination to regain his prior functioning. That determination is reflected in the tremendous amount of work he invested in "doing battle" with his illness, as delineated in chapter 4, "Reading.".

Weinstein specifies in his Introduction that the four audiences for this book are the general aging population, stroke victims and survivors, caregivers, and students in college speech therapy. They can learn from this stroke victim and survivor the difficult realities that people who suffer strokes have to endure and how those hard realities can be surmounted. Weinstein also provides check lists for stroke survivors, and their spouses and 'friends, to help them deal more effectively with the consequences of stroke and aphasia. The author has a made a major contribution to the fields of stroke, aphasia, and patient rehabilitation.

By Edna M. Babbitt, M.Ed., CCC-SLP, BC-ANCDS
Research Speech-Language Pathologist
Rehabilitation Institute of Chicago
Center for Aphasia Research & Treatment

Readers of *My Stroke* by Dr. Weinstein will follow his recovery after a stroke and diagnosis of aphasia. It is not an easy journey to take with him as he shares his emotional highs and lows. In reading his experiences, I recall the stories of many of my former patients. Through his writing, we are able to walk step-by-step through his recovery and discover how he learns to live with aphasia. He is honest in sharing not only his negative feelings but also his triumphs, successes and the deep love felt for those close to him. He writes in depth about his experience with speech therapy and the exercises which helped him. Each chapter starts with a review and ends with checklists or helpful hints for readers (both people with aphasia and their family or caregivers) to take away. Speech therapists will gain insight into what it is like to live with aphasia on a daily basis. It is important to read stories about living with aphasia, such as Dr. Weinstein's, as many people living with aphasia are not able to talk and express their thoughts. Dr. Weinstein's motivation to keep working and moving forward is an inspiration. He writes the thoughts of many people with aphasia which are unspoken.

Introduction

It has been a cathartic exercise for me to chronicle and sequence the major milestones of my stroke in detail, from stroke victim with great disabilities to stroke survivor coping with daily tasks so that I could go on with my life.

This book is a case study about the fifteen months of my life after my stroke and the journey that I traveled to become what I am now. When I entered Transitions of Long Island in February 2002 I had had an embolic cerebrovascular accident with severe aphasia. I couldn't speak, read, write, sing or do arithmetic. By the time I graduated from Transitions of Long Island, in May 2003, I had re-acquired some of the skills I needed to use to speak with my family and friends, read books slowly and make some change in stores. Today I am able to make business presentations, read classics, and write articles and this book. But I am not "whole". I still have some problems with my speech. I read slowly. I stutter periodically. I can't find words to express my thoughts. I make some tense errors in both writing and speaking. I make grammatical mistakes also.

There is a wealth of information in this book but it is not a handbook and it is not proscriptive primarily because a stroke is different for each person. The value of this study is in the details and the real feel that comes from the interaction of these particulars. That is true when the reader comes upon the educational jargon -terminology, domains and percentiles- administrated for neuropsychological tests. The results of my tests differ from other stroke victims' but the reader would have a better understanding of the process used to monitor the growth of any stroke victim by the professional staff. This concept would hold true when I walk you through my interface with my computer as I re-learned to write. Obviously, other stroke victims and survivors have other ways to improve their writing skills. But the reader would know the feel of the painstaking task of writing.

There are four audiences for this book. This book is intended for the:

1. general aging population who are scrupulously aware of the growing numbers of stroke victims,
2. stroke victims and survivors,
3. caregivers, and
4. students in college speech therapy programs.

There is information about insurance companies, neuropsychological progress reports, speech therapists and pathologists, other patients, supportive groups, business issues, travel, vacations, holidays, driving and eating in restaurants and diners. There is the give and take between me and my family and my speech therapist. There is raw anger and fear, infantile behavior, growth, emotional and physical stress, mercurial ups and downs, privacy and dignity. There are predators and good Samaritans. This book understands the pressure placed on caregivers.

This book is based on my experiences as a stroke victim and stroke survivor. These two terms have different meaning to me. As a stroke victim I was not able to communicate except in the most elementary ways. At best there were a few words, maybe no more than ten words if that, that I could say with certainty daily. At worst I made sounds, as I tried to mouth words, or made dog like barks to get my thoughts to others.

When I think of a stroke survivor, such as me, I think of the physical illness, a disease, which is permanent and the severe aphasia which doesn't have to be severe or permanent for my life. There are medicines and exercise regiments to help me to control the disease. But the fight against severe aphasia and the loss of speech, reading, writing, singing and arithmetic is essentially up to the gods, luck, discipline and hard work.

My speech pathologist, Peggy Kramer, suggested that I might want to write an essay about my stroke. She and I understood that I might find this to be painful. Peggy casually mentioned to me that a couple of women wrote a book on their brain injuries. Obviously, if others could write a book surely I could write an essay maybe a book. As a result of writing this book it became even clearer to me that Peggy Kramer saved my spirit and soul the day that I entered Transitions of Long Island.

There are two parts of this book. One part, Chapters 1-3, deals with stroke victims. Stroke victims may not be able to read this book but a caregiver can. Part two, Chapters 4-6, deals with stroke survivors. This is for the stroke survivor and the caregiver. A stroke survivor is able to read at least a little bit. Each chapter starts with a preview and a list of the issues that will be discussed in the chapter. At the end of each chapter there are check lists for stroke survivors and caregivers.

Chapter 1: February 2002 - *The Days After My Stroke* deals with my anger and fear in the hospital, frustration with my insurance company and the love of my family.

Chapter 2: March 2002 - *Baseline Information Shares the First Month of my Rehabilitation*, the individuality of my stroke, the re-regimentation of my days, rehabilitation at Transitions of Long Island, my supporters, issues of dignity and humiliation and my new role within in my family.

Chapter 3: April 2002-July 2002 - *My Unfolding Passage on the Continuum from Stroke Victim to Stroke Survivor* provides information about my neuropsychological report as a framework to understand my accomplishments, as limited as they were, in different areas of my life.

Chapter 4: April-July 2002 – *Reading* spells out my struggle to relearn to read, benefits derived as I read three books by the end of the summer and my effort to become an outgoing person.

Chapter 5: August-October 2002 – *I Could* occupies three months of my life, the uphill struggles and growth that I observed in myself as I went on vacation with my family, reestablished my consultancies, and continued to improve my reading, relearn writing and sing songs.

Chapter 6: November 2002 –May 2003 – *The Battle for My Dignity* deals with the last seven months of my rehabilitation, the changes in my relationships with family and friends, travel to Puerto Rico, overcoming abusive behavior by law agencies, the insurance company and the joy and pride that comes from reading.

This book takes a look at what goes into the spirit and soul of a stroke victim, the nuances that are not spoken about in cursory workshops and never detailed in lectures. There is the emotional throbbing pain and accomplishments, as modest as there are day in and day out and the issues and events that affect the stroke victim and perhaps you too. If you are a spouse you will see yourself in the vignettes that are integrated through this book. There are streams of consciousness and free flow thoughts wrapped throughout each chapter. These allow you, the stroke victim and the spouse, to see the way that real life intermixes with both of you. The idea is that you may see something that is important to you that you didn't think about before and it may help you.

There are many wonderful organizations and agencies, such as the American Stroke Association, National Institute on Deafness and Other Communication Disorders, American Speech-Language-Hearing-Association, Brain Injury Association of America, Easter Seals, Inc., and The National Aphasia Association. There are many technical books about strokes, aphasia and speech-language-hearing for the approximately one million people who have aphasia. They don't share the day to day subtleties in real time world situations for the stroke victim and the spouse or significant other, children, family and friends. This book does.

Acknowledgements

In the past when I wrote nonfictional books I would end my acknowledgements by thanking my family for allowing me to spend the time I needed to write a book. Not this time. This is because my wife, Dale, and my family, especially my son Jeff and his wife my daughter-in-law, Anne, were integral in every part of this narrative.

Dale cared, nourished, cheered, and cried for me every day. She loved me with an intensity, part passion and part despair, that surpassed any love that I could imagine, a love that I couldn't spell out in a thousand words. She protected me and heard me when most of the world thought I was silent. Dale edited large parts of my manuscript and never tried to change the essence of my story even though it was painful for her to read my thoughts.

My love for Jeff is overwhelming. He was and is a tower of comfort for me. I am reassured by his integrity, optimism and respect for all people but most of all by his love of his wife and his two children Alison and Jessica. Anne is more than a daughter-in-law. She is the perfect partner for Jeff and a demonstrative, compassionate, witty woman who always had and has time for me when I call and that is about twice a week. I got lucky when Jeff married Anne. I know that I wouldn't have recuperated so quickly without their love, encouragement, and concern.

My granddaughters, Alison and Jessica, were the reasons that I worked as hard as I did to relearn to read and speak. They were my motivations. I wanted to read to them and share thoughts with them. I know that I made progress because I saw them in my mind even though I didn't know that at the time but I was there.

This book pays homage to Peggy Kramer, my speech therapist at <u>Transitions of Long Island</u>, without who I would have died spiritually and emotionally. Instead I thrived. She taught me to speak, read, and write. She nurtured me every day in multiple ways. We laughed and cried. We worked and played. We tried and failed and tried again and succeeded. She pushed me every day. My silence gave way to words and laughter and personhood. She seriously encouraged me in my hopes. Peggy was part of my day every day for fifteen months. This book wouldn't have been written without Peggy.

I'm appreciative to my good friend Pierre Woog, Ph.D, who edited the draft of this book. He and I "talked" almost daily from the first day I was released from the hospital until I was discharged from <u>Transitions of Long Island</u> and so he was knowledgeable about the major issues and events that were covered in this book.

People in the Book

My biological family	
Dale	My wife
Jeffrey (Jeff)	My oldest son
Anne	My daughter-in-law, Jeff's wife
Alison	My oldest granddaughter, Anne and Jeff's daughter
Jessica	Anne and Jeff's youngest daughter and my second oldest granddaughter
Robert	My middle son
Erick	My youngest son
Professional staff at North Shore University Hospital	
Dr. Stanley Katz	Chairman of Cardiology
Dr. Rothstein	Neurologist
Professional staff at Transitions of Long Island (part of North Shore University Hospital)	
Peggy Kramer	My primary speech therapist.
Deena Shein	My first speech therapist
Deborah Benson, Ph.D	Director of Transitions of Long Island
Friends	
Pierre Woog, Ph.D	Former Education Dean and a good friend.
Fred	Health Gym Store owner
Lou	Patron at Fred's store
Patricia Mc Leod	Assistant Superintendent at Middletown New York
Hannah Hill	Teacher at the Roosevelt School District

Jeff's In-Laws	
Mary	Anne's mother
Marvin	Anne's father
Karen	Anne's sister
David	Anne's bother-in-law
Susie	Anne's sister
Mark	Anne's bother-in-law
My blended family	
Mark	Dale's son
Dana	Mark's wife
Lily	Mark and Dana's daughter. She calls me grandpa and I consider her my granddaughter
Jill	Dale's daughter
Julian	Jill's husband
Tod	Dale's brother
Stephanie	Tod's significant other
Extended family for Passover	
Bernie	My first cousin
Connie	Bernie's wife
Dorothy	My first cousin, Bernie's sister
Karsten	Dorothy's ex son-in-law
Seth	Bernie's son

Stroke Victim and Stroke Survivor: Fifteen Months in Transitions of Long Island. February 2002- May 2003

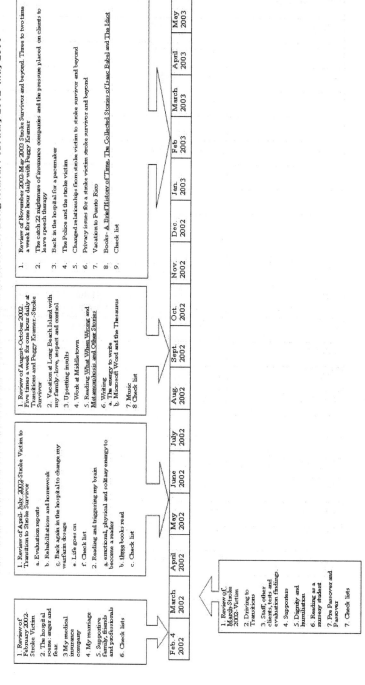

Timeline: Feb. 4 2002 | March 2002 | April 2002 | May 2002 | June 2002 | July 2002 | Aug. 2002 | Sept. 2002 | Oct. 2002 | Nov. 2002 | Dec. 2002 | Jan. 2003 | Feb 2003 | March 2003 | April 2003 | May 2003

Box 1:
1. Review of February 2002- Stroke Victim
2. The hospital scene: anger and fear
3 My medical insurance company
4. My marriage
5. Supportive family, friends and professionals
6. Check lists

Box (March 2002):
1. Review of March-Stroke 2002-Victim
2. Driving to Transitions
3. Staff, other clients, tests and evaluation findings.
4. Supporters
5. Dignity and humiliation
6. Reading as a nursery student
7. Pre Passover and Passover
7. Check lists

Box (April- July 2002):
1. Review of April- July 2002-Stroke Victim to Transition to Stroke Survivor
   a. Evaluation reports
   b. Rehabilitation and homework
   c. Back again in the hospital to change my warfarin dosage
   e. Life goes on
   f. Check list
2. Reading and triggering my brain
   a. emotional, physical and solitary energy to become a reader
   b. these books read
   c. Check list

Box (Aug.- Sept. 2002):
1. Review of August-October 2002. Five times a week for one hour daily at Transitions and Peggy Kramer.-Stroke Survivor
2. Vacation at Long Beach Island with my family- love, respect and control
3. Upsetting insults
4. Work at Middletown
5. Reading What When Wrong and Metamorphosis and Other Stories
6. Writing
   a. The energy to write
   b. Microsoft Word and the Thesaurus
7. Music
8 Check list

Box (Nov. 2002- May 2003):
1. Review of November 2002-May 2003 Stroke Survivor and beyond. Three to two time a week for one hour daily with Peggy Kramer
2. The catch 22 nightmare of insurance companies and the pressure placed on clients to leave speech therapy
3. Back in the hospital for a pacemaker
4. The Police and the stroke victim
5. Changed relationships from stroke victim to stroke survivor and beyond
6. Privacy issues for a stroke victim stroke survivor and beyond
7. Vacation to Puerto Rico
8. Books- A Brief History of Time, The Collected Stories of Isaac Babel and The Idiot
9. Check list

1

Chapter 1: February 2002
The Days After My Stroke

Preview

This chapter gives you a realistic picture of the metamorphosis that happens in a stroke. You will see how fragile I was after my stroke and the supportive groups that helped me. Remember, your stroke victim is unique. There are a variety of factors that your stroke victim and you cannot control. But there are many things that the stroke victim can do to better improve his life. You need to use your strength to deal with your insurance company and this chapter gives you an idea of the problems. As Cervantes said 400 years ago "Forewarned, forearmed; to be prepared is half the victory." Now take on the insurance companies.

What this chapter gives to you in a first person account is the mindset of a stroke victim:

◊ Consumed with anger and fear before one is able to speak, read or write.
◊ Your insurance company and your marriage.
◊ Supportive family, friends and professionals.

The hospital: anger and fear, family and acquaintances, and the nothingness in my soul

The second I woke up from my stroke that day in the hospital I was frightened even before I uttered any words. It was similar to Monet's Haystack. There was a pale hue; there were changing lights. The color was gray purple. It seemed to me that I was not visible. I could not see out of my bed and others could not see me. It seemed to me that I was a part of a vague light and I could be a fragment that would not be perceived. In a moment I knew that I could not speak, read, or write. I could not communicate. The nurses spoke to my wife Dale and son Jeff. Discussions were with my son and wife and the doctors, nurses and my business associates. Suddenly, I knew that I could not talk.

I could not talk to myself. In those moments I was a non-identity. I wanted to die at least I thought so although maybe not. I remembered that I cried. In a primordial yell, howl and moan I told my son that I wanted to die if I could not speak, read or write. These moments, these were frightening seconds and minutes, this torment. I was a pale tone, not seen or heard or felt.

Yet in midst of this I remembered that I had a vague thought. Jeff was wearing a brown leather lambskin jacket. I never saw him in it before. I smiled to myself. I never thought of Jeff as a guy who wore leather jackets. Than I thought it was nice. I was able to think this without a single word.

I had always thought that I would have on my lips the names of my wife, Dale, sons Jeff, Robert and Erick, my granddaughters Alison and Jessica and my daughter-in-law Anne when I died and maybe a prayer also. I wanted to see them just as I died, with my last breath. But now I couldn't say Dale. I couldn't say Jeff. I couldn't say Robert. I couldn't say Erick. I couldn't say Anne. But I cried because I couldn't say Alison and Jessica. I sobbed because Jeff shed tears for himself and me when I couldn't remember their names much less verbalize them. I felt so sad so angry. I wanted to help Jeff.

The only thing that I knew was that I felt sorry because I hurt my son, Jeff, and wife, Dale, especially Jeff because of my agony. I will never do that again. I learned how much he loved me. When my first wife died at 33 years of age after a long illness Jeff and I would sleep in my bed periodically right after my wife and his mother, died. He was nine years old. I knew that Jeff was comforted by me but I never knew whether Jeff knew that he comforted me in the days and weeks that followed.

In the days following my stroke I felt the same calm and composure when I saw Jeff's face and gentle eyes. I knew that he needed me to get better so that he could slowly face my death in the future.

4

I was in the Horton Medical Center from February 4th to 7th and in North Shore University Hospital from the 7th to 12th. I remember some things about these times in these hospitals. Dale and Jeff saw me from the time I was in the Horton Medical Center. My wife and I lived in Nassau County, a good 100 miles away from the Horton Medical Center in Middletown, New York. Jeff lived in New Jersey about 120 miles away from Middletown.

Dale was an elementary teacher. She taught science. She was a conscientious and concerned teacher. I remembered that she would be overwhelmed by my stroke, and she would worry about her classes. She would not want to worry about the classes but I knew that she could not help herself. I wanted her to see me, love me, and I wanted her to go back to her friends in school to comfort herself. I knew these thoughts. I did.

I had my stroke when I worked as a consultant in the Middletown School District. Most of my time was spent in the Maple Hill Elementary School. Some of the teachers from the Middletown School District visited me for a couple minutes. They were Lea and Sue. I could not say their names or remember them. The Maple Hill School's nurse saw me one time. She diagnosed my stroke when I sat in the principal's office waiting to talk with the Principal, Paula Amaditz. The Assistant Superintendent, Pat McLeod, spent a couple of hours daily with my wife and son. Periodically, one of them said something to me. My wife and son answered for me but Jeff always looked at me with such feelings to see if I could answer by myself.

Within one or two days it was clear that I was asked by the nurses to lead a life of quiet desperation, a life of resignation. I was not able to say these thoughts. It was in my mind. It was obscured, vague in my mind, but it was there. The hospital staffs were nice people. My wife has said they were pleasant to her and Jeff. But my thoughts were my thoughts.

When I think of this period I think of trees as skeletons, with weak trunks and worn out outer bark. There weren't different colors in the trees in the Appalachians forests. There wasn't a cacophony of sights in the fall colors found in oaks, spruces, pines, beeches, elms, and mahogany. Yet my soul fought and I saw periodically bright reds but also gray greens.

One of my thoughts was red hot with malice and fretful about my dignity and my essence. I was trained, trained to be like a prisoner, incarcerated and enslaved, to be a prisoner who feels some kinship to the guard who watches him. In One Flew Over The Cuckoo's Nest Chief Bromden writes chronic patients are kept in the hospital, "to keep them from walking around the street giving the product a bad name..." Stroke victims are never heard. They just are enraged because hospital staffs don't want to take the time to allow them to try to say a letter or a word. It is not time efficient.

At the same time there were gray green pictures of old helpless people walking two by two led by nurses or no one just a long line going nowhere. There were lines of young children, young and old women and men going nowhere from nowhere, always in pajamas, colorless pajamas. They were not able to pray or hate because their words were not in their mouths or brains. People never said another word to another person. Each second a person keeled over and died. No one stopped to help or comfort. There was no one to testify about his existence. No one knew his thoughts or hopes after the stroke.

Three days after I was admitted to Horton Medical Center, February 4, 2002, my cardiologist in Long Island, Dr. Stanley Katz, Chairman of Cardiology, moved me to North Shore University Hospital. In addition to medical reasons I felt safer with Dr. Katz. I trusted him. The facility seemed newer, more advanced, and also personal. I owed a debt to Middletown hospital and its doctors and nurses. But I needed to see Dr. Katz. I needed to see my wife daily and not worry about her traveling 100 miles to see me. I needed to see Jeff and not worry that my daughter-in-law and granddaughters would miss him when he came to visit.

Unfortunately, my sons Robert and Erick came to see me but I don't remember when. Nor did I recall Anne's visit. Anne was and is the best daughter-in-law period. She made my son happy. She was and is a good partner to him. She made me and Dale welcomed to their home. She gives us unlimited time with Alison and Jessica. She was and is my daughter. Nor did I remember the visit of my stepson, Mark, and his wife, Dana. I didn't remember any one else.

The godless bureaucracy of the medical insurance company and my marriage

After five days in <u>North Shore University Hospital</u>, on the day of my discharge, a social worker gave us a list of numbers of speech pathologists that could help me. She gave us a list. She didn't talk to any speech pathologists for me. She didn't explain the procedures to get my insurance provider, <u>Empire</u>, to move quickly so that I could get in to a speech program after the hospital stay.

When I came home on February 12th all hell broke loose and I thought that my marriage would end. As soon as we came home I wanted to call the speech pathologists. Dale called a bunch of speech pathologists. They were private practices. There were a few agencies or organizations. Dale and I found out that we needed to first get permission from my insurance company before we could talk with pathologists especially sole practice pathologists. None of the six or so pathologists wanted to help us to deal with the red tape called <u>Empire</u>.

I have had difficulty buying gum much less shoes much less a suit much less a car. How was I to hire a speech pathologist? Did I know what a speech pathologist did and how would I know whether they did their job well? How would I know whether the speech pathologist had success with people like me? After all I couldn't say a vowel much less a word. <u>Empire</u> didn't help me in this way.

One of the suggested places was <u>Transitions of Long Island</u>. Dale phoned. A secretary told her that it would take weeks or months before my insurer, <u>Empire</u>, would agree to pay <u>Transitions of Long Island</u> for speech and or cognitive therapy. Dale said it would take some time to get in to <u>Transitions of Long Island</u>. I yelled. Why didn't she push? Why didn't she allow me to talk? If she couldn't do that then I would do it myself. After all it was my life. Let me talk if you…All the time I growled because I could not speak. However, I was able to get my feeling across to Dale.

The only words that I could say were "fuck it" and "shit". At the hospital I couldn't remember to say "Dale" even though she and I worked on her name. My frustration exploded and I yelled out "Jesus Christ". Dale said that was a start so I called her "Jesus Christ" whenever. So I had five words in my vocabulary to show anger and frustration. I was able to yell and motion. The more I wanted to talk to Dale or secretaries I gnarled grumbled or roared. There were sounds but no words except "shit" and "fuck it" and a word or two that came out of my mouth and I couldn't repeat it if my life depended on it. There were gargled sounds but no real words. There were wolf sounds but no real words. By the time it was 5 P.M. we were drained, panicked, and dismayed.

I feared. I feared about my speech. I feared about my right leg. I feared about my eye. I feared about my writing. I feared. I feared about another stroke. I feared about my heart. I feared.

I feared that I had to free Dale. She looked strong but she was terrified. Her first husband died. She raised her son and daughter. She made due, barely. I thought that she must have thought that she might have to live a life a quiet desperation too. I could not endure that for her and me. She needed to go to the beach on sunny days during the spring, summer and fall. She needed to walk the boardwalk or on the sand in Long Beach or Jones Beach on cold sunny winter days. She needed to spend time with her friends, go to lunch or dinner with them, work out at the yoga center once or twice a week, go to the movies or the museums or the Aquarium in Coney Island once in a while and spend time with Alison and Jessica. I thought that Dale was like a museum white Russian Faberge porcelain egg, hard on the outside and so delicate in side that she would break.

That day I loved her and wanted her and needed her. Yet I was afraid that she would crack under the pressure that I would put on her. I needed to struggle to survive, to fight for my life and I feared that Dale would snap. I thought that Dale thought that she would break.

She was not capable to confront the quagmire of the Empire bureaucracy and me. She told me that day that she would try to help me as much as she could. I knew that she would but I knew that it was time limited; not because of Dale but because of me. I didn't know how I would fight but I knew it. I would fight. I was afraid that it was a no win situation. On one side there was Dale's gentleness and desire to help me. There was another side covered by my frustration and my wrath. That evening after all the calls were made Dale and I hugged and loved and cried and touched eyes, fingered tears, fondled lips, rubbed ears, and stroked noses, and we wailed.

The next few days were a tragic comedy. Dale was able to connect with the people at Transitions of Long Island. They agreed to see me and to evaluate me at once. That was testimony to Dale's push and the secretaries' sensitivities at Transitions of Long Island. They knew how to talk with her. They put her in touch with Peggy Kramer, Coordinator, and Speech-Language Therapy Services. Mrs. Kramer told Dale to bring me over to Transitions of Long Island the next morning so that Mrs. Kramer could evaluate my speech and cognitive problems.

9

I have little memory of this evaluation and the details of results come from a report, <u>Initial Speech-Language Evaluation,</u> written by Peggy Kramer Coordinator, Speech-Language Therapy Services at <u>Transitions of Long Island</u>. Mrs. Kramer administered the <u>Minnesota Test for Different Diagnosis of Aphasia</u> to me to assess my current strengths and weaknesses in auditory, visual and reading, speech and language, visuomotor and writing skill areas. This evaluation demonstrated my strengths in auditory discrimination and recognition and visual discrimination and recognition.

Evaluation Finding

	February 13, 2002
1.0 Auditory Disturbances	
1.1 recognize common words	18/18
1.2 discriminate paired words	24/24
1.3 recognize letters	21/26
1.4 identify items named serially	6/6
1.5 answered simple questions correctly	14/15
1.6 followed oral directions	6/10
1.7 asked yes/no questions related to a verbally presented paragraph	5/6
1.8 repeat 2 and 3 digit numbers	Correct
1.9 repeat sentences	0/6
2.0 Visual and reading subtests	
2.1 match form to pictures	5/5
2.2 match letters to pictures	20/20
2.3 match words to pictures	32/32
2.4 match printed to spoken words	32/32
2.5 comprehended sentences based on yes/no format	14/15
2.6 yes/no questions related to paragraph	6/8
2.7 reading words	1/15
2.8 reading sentences	0/30
3.0 Speech and Language Disturbance	
3.1 imitated appropriate phonation,	Correct

tongue movements, palatal movement and pharyngeal movements given a model by the clinician	
3.2 appropriate protrusion, retraction and lateral movement of his tongue	Correct
3.3 repeat monosyllable words with difficulty noted towards the end of the list with blends (e.g. /sk/, /st/, /sch/, and /tr/).	26/32
3.4 repeat phrases	4/20
3.5 counting to 20 and reciting the days of the week	Correct
3.6 completing sentences and answering simple questions related to using common objects	4/8
3.7 asked to produce sentences given a stimulus word	0/6
3.8 describing a picture	0/6
3.9 name picture	4/20
4.0 Visuomotor and Writing Disturbances	
4.1 copy Greek	5/5
4.2 copy numbers	20/20
4.3 reproduce a drawing of a wheel with spokes	Correct
4.4 reproduce letters	18/18
4.5 writing letters to dictation	16/26
4.6 written spelling	2/10
4.7 oral spelling	0/10

Overall, I had significant difficulty with auditory recalls. My visual and reading tests indicated inconsistent articulation, general slurring, marked slowness and the substitution of words.

The word definition and retelling a paragraph sub-tests were not administered due to the more difficult nature of the tasks and my aphasia. Sub-tests targeting production of written sentences, writing sentences to dictation and writing a paragraph were not administered due to the level of difficulty involved. Also, time did not permit for the numerical relations and arithmetic processes sub-tests.

The bottom line was that I had moderate to severe deficits in receptive language areas. That included auditory retention span, word finding, following verbal directions (2 step), digit repetition, sentence repetition, reading rate, and oral reading of words and sentences. I had severe deficits in expressive language areas. That included repetition of monosyllables (words), repetition of phrases, completion of sentences, expression of ideas, production of sentences, descriptive language, and picture naming. I had severe difficulty with written language when asked to spell words in written and oral forms, and produce written sentences.

At the end of the evaluation Mrs. Kramer told Dale that Transitions of Long Island would file the papers to start the process to get Empire to pay for Transitions of Long Island services. She did not know whether Empire would pay for all services that I needed or the number of weeks of services. Mrs. Kramer said that Empire was a good insurance company. Peggy Kramer said that Dale would have to talk to Empire and it might take a month or two before Empire would agree to pay the cost to Transitions of Long Island. Dale told Peggy that I had to be in Transitions of Long Island at once so that I could start my rehabilitation.

My experiences with Empire, my insurer, seem to be a scene from Charlie Chaplin's Modern Times with cogs and angst caused by vicious technological innovations especially computers and voice messages. Empire had one of those answering machines, one that didn't cite the specific department needed much less the specific person who could help me. Also, Empire didn't train its staff from my point of view to be tolerant with the stroke victims and their families.

Dale called Empire. The Empire bureaucracy was made of people who shut down their collective minds. At the times that Dale called them they had idyllic empty-headedness. She was first asked a series of questions than she was transferred to another person. That person asked the same questions but didn't have any answer. Dale was on the phone for three hours the first day. On the second day there was more of the same.

Dale was a gentle person and she didn't want to push the Empire people hard. She was frustrated but she was a gentlewoman. I was furious. I was enraged because Dale didn't listen to me when I tried to tell her what to say. I was livid because I was not able to help myself and I could not remember my thoughts nor was I able to form a word. I could not even say "I" or "is". I just wanted to help myself and I couldn't.

Then after three days Dale used me as a resource to help myself. Once Dale found a person that knew something about strokes and programs I helped myself. I roared and bellowed in the phone. Dale then told the person that I had a Ph.D and that it was imperative for me to get in to a speech program. Finally, a Ms. Anderson, a supervisor type woman, bright, courteous, a mentsh walked the paperwork through. It took a couple of weeks but Ms. Anderson assured Dale and I that Empire would pay for my speech rehabilitation for six months and they would determine my rehabilitation after that. Eventually, Empire paid Transitions of Long Island for me for fifteen months.

Supportive Family, Friends and Professionals

In the midst of this fright and anger there was a shinning glimmer of hope although I didn't see all of it right away especially my support group of family, friends and professionals.

One February Friday morning Anne came over with my youngest granddaughter, Jessica. Jessica was about twelve months old. She was beautiful. She had brown hair, a cute small face and eyes of brown pools. Anne came over to make sure that I could use my software program and folders. She was to make files for four schools that I was supposed to enter data for in a time-on-task program. Anne probably thought I could help but I was useless. I didn't remember the name of my program or where it was in the computer. I felt terrible that Anne had to come over and that Jessica had to go through this ordeal for me.

Dale watched Jessica when Jessica was awakened. Anne and I sat on the floor. Anne looked and found the program and copied the program to three separate folders. I remembered that I was irritated with myself because I put this burden on Anne. She must have been upset because she knew that she had to get Alison, my oldest granddaughter, before school ended and that would be a 90 minutes drive. I also knew that I made her and Dale nervous.

My agony was evident. I believed that Anne must have felt like she had to walk on eggs because of my inability to show her the program and my groans of frustration. In reality I was very overjoyed. Anne helped me to see an inkling of a star, a place I wanted to be. After four or five hours Anne finished.

I was the luckiest father-in-law in the whole wide world. I remembered that I cried because of Anne and because I had a chance to do work. Also, I cried sometimes just because.

Once Anne developed the files and she went home I tried to use my program and enter data. It was difficult. I couldn't remember even one number. I was not able to say numbers greater than nine. I had to look at a number and then I had to input data. To do that I had to look at the number and I had to find the number on the keyboard. By the time I looked at the number keys I forgot the number. It was more difficult to input data for tens and above. If the data sheet for a teacher had 15 minutes for a standard or performance indicator I would first input a 5 and then I would input a 1before the 5 so that the number was 15. Once I knew that I could input data, no matter how slowly, I believed that I could finish the project for Maple Hill.

During my stay in <u>North Shore University Hospital</u> Dale spoke the Paula Amaditz, the Principal and told her to send all the data sheets from the teachers to be inputted. Once Anne copied all my files and made new files and I was able to input data. Dale called Patricia McLeod and told her that I could finish my time-on-task audit of the delivery of standards and performance indicators. Pat said that she would take a chance on me for the rest of the academic year for Maple Hill but she would hold off for the three other schools. Within two weeks of my coming home my computer program was usable and I had work to do.

My friend, Pierre Woog, Ph.D, was in touch with Dale from the first day I was in the hospital at <u>Horton Medical Center</u>. Pierre and his wife Kendall helped Dale to reduce the disjointed pace that happens in these moments. They lived about 30-40 minutes from Middletown. I had rented a car from <u>Enterprise</u> in West Hempstead. When Dale and Jeff came to see me they had to deal with the rented car. Dale called <u>Enterprise</u> and they waved the fees if she could get the rented car to <u>Enterprise</u> in Middletown. The next day Pierre and Kendall drove to Middletown. They took the car the <u>Enterprise</u>. It reduced Dale's stress and allowed her to deal with the numerous hospital issues, work issues and personal issues that consumed her.

Pierre told me about my speech condition when I came home from <u>North Shore University Hospital</u>. You see Pierre called me every morning like clockwork at about 7:10 a.m. the time when his wife went to work. Pierre prides himself as an active listener. An active listener focuses attention of the speaker, in this case me. I could be glib at this point about any professor who thinks that he is an active listener but I know that Pierre was genuinely worried about my physical condition.

Pierre and I always fought on all kinds of issues since I worked for him at Adelphi University when he was Dean of Education. As we got older we became feisty old cocks. We enjoyed the intellectual battles and the stories about families. We supported each other. So whatever Pierre said

I would have to take his reflections as pretty accurate. Pierre said that he didn't understand my speech although there were a couple of words that he might have understood. Also, I stuttered. The talks were short maybe two to five minutes for the first month. That was a friend.

Conclusion

In retrospect there were many changes that happened so quickly; changes of maturity, death and birth and brilliance and ignorance and consciousness. Dylan Thomas cautions "Do not go gentle into that good night, Old age should burn and rave at close of day; Rage, rage against the dying of the light." How does one rage against the dying of the light when one doesn't know the light is off?

Checklists

Victim needs to:

1. Try to get all the sleep possible so that in the morning the stroke victim can give hell to the hospital staff.
2. Try hard to talk or babble or growl so that people know that you are also a person.

Family members need to:

1. Get a good night sleep after you see your spouse or parent or child.
2. Write out the name of tasks that need to be tackled right away:
    ◊ Doctors
    ◊ Insurance companies
    ◊ Employer and colleagues
    ◊ Other family members
    ◊ Friends
3. Make sure that you have your spouse's, parent's or children's insurance information in detail.
4. Encourage the stroke victim to interact with you and the nurses and doctors.

Chapter 2: March 2002 - Baseline Information
The First Month of My Rehabilitation

Review

This chapter gives you a picture of my first four weeks at <u>Transitions of Long Island,</u> the assiduous efforts by Peggy and Deena and all the staff to nurse me back to health as a "whole" person, the supplementary help given to me by my wife, Dale, who cared for me twenty-four hours seven days a week, family, especially Jeff and Anne, who called me daily and visited me a number of times in those weeks, and friends, such as Pierre and Fred, and my new role within my family as showed at Pesach (Passover).

I was infantized by the English language and the words and thoughts and subtleties that the language conveys. The English language shed an ominous gray shadow on me and changed my world. I ceased to be my own person, with my own space and personality. Instead I was a hyphenated person a Don-Dale or Dale-Don. My thoughts came from Dale's mouth not mine and her behaviors became mine also. There was no privacy. Dale went to the doctors with me and answered questions for me and gave my orders to waitress in restaurants and diners.

There were assaults by others on my personhood, my dignity, my respect and my violent fits of self pity.

At the same time in the same moments I saw Dale's beauty, her green-blue eyes, the soul of her pain, and the fragile fibers that make the spirit of Dale. The gods gave me Jeff and they allowed me to see him grow into a mature, sensitive, caring husband, father and person. And there was the beauty, smiles and hopes in my life that were named Anne, Alison and Jessica.

The fact that I was able to write this account of my stroke means that I was able to store in my brain the events, perceptions and thoughts that I write. During the month of

March, 2002, on a continuum of 0-100, I probably achieved a grade of 1 in speaking .5 in reading and .2 in writing. However, I was able to have my brain accumulate a vast conglomeration of daily happening; a potpourri that I didn't even know was in my brain.

This chapter gives you the frame of mind for a stroke victim. It gives you a first person account of a one month stroke victim in your home. Expect stroke victims to have:

- ◊ Mercurial ups and downs in short order
- ◊ Needs to express the most simplistic sounds and words and gestures by himself
- ◊ Desires to show himself and the caregiver that he can do something by himself so let him do it
- ◊ Time away from his house where he can look at old and new people and places
- ◊ Cravings for his family, a family that makes him comfortable
- ◊ Needs that can be satisfied only by his granddaughters nearness to him and kissing them on their heads

Driving to <u>Transitions of Long Island</u>

This was a story about luck. It was luck that I had the best education in the whole world and it was luck that I worked out two to four days a week every week before I had my stroke. There was a stroke of luck that I had the best doctors to help me to recover and the best speech therapists to help me to become "whole" and the best physical therapists too. I had a great support system of family and friends as well as discipline, planning, and strategies but most of it was luck.

Dale planned a troop movement to prepare me for my first day in <u>Transitions of Long Island</u>. We went to the <u>T-Mobile</u> store to buy two cell phones. We knew that it would be essential to have a way for both of us to make contact. Dale showed me how to dial phone numbers and to answer the cell phone. She drove me to <u>Transitions of Long</u>

Island so that I would be familiar with the streets to Transitions of Long Island. The thought was to allow me to feel comfortable in a taxi and have some control over my life. Dale wrote the taxi's phone number for me.

Troop movements were nothing compared to the real battles. The taxi, Ollie, came late. Dale had left for work at 7 a.m. At about 7:45 a.m., I started looking for the taxi. It was suppose to arrive at my house at 8:00 a.m. Every minute or so I got out of my chair in the dining room to look out of the window for the taxi. At 8:00 a.m. I panicked. There was no taxi. In some ways every time I went to the window I thought for a tiny second the vehicles in the distance on Dogwood Avenue were taxis. There was a mirage, a suburban oasis filled with taxis. My thirst for Ollie' taxi was real but there were no taxis. I couldn't reach a taxi. I could see time but I could not say time.

I dialed the telephone number and called Ollie's taxi company. The dispatcher on the other side of the phone could not understand my sounds and then my yelling. The more I was frustrated the more I shrieked. The more I shrieked the more I knew that I had to call Dale at her school to tell her to get the taxi over to me quickly. The more that I required Dale's help the more I felt infantized. As soon as I got on the phone Dale knew that I had a problem with the taxi company. It was one of those things that she knew at once. Dale called the taxi company and the dispatcher sent a taxi a couple of minutes later. This routine lasted for one five day week.

There was no mark on me to indicate that I was a North American or a stroke victim. I had no conversational ability in any language at the time. Some of these drivers must have assumed that I was from some other country and they continued talking to me. I liked the sounds of their voices. It cost about $25 each way or a total of $250 for the week. Subsequently, I found out that Nassau County had a Bus Access transportation program in place. I could have taken the Bus Access from my home to Transitions of Long Island

and back but it would have consumed a lot of my time. Unfortunately, public officials seem to believe that handicapped, retirees and poor people have unlimited time to come and go.

During this time Dale took me to my doctors-Dr. Rothstein, an earthy brilliant neurologist, and Dr. Katz, somewhere between a Titan and a product of a god and a human. These doctors indicated that I was fit to drive. They signed the MVD document that I could drive. They warned Dale and me that I might get lost at first. We thought that was no big deal. We live on an island. As long as I didn't cross a bridge I could be found easily or I could find my house.

This was a very important moment to both me and Dale. I was able to be more independent day in and day out. I was able to go and come at my own pace. I could decide to stay home or I could go to the mall or the park or to the museum or physical therapy. Yet there were a number of steps that had to be mastered including driving to Transitions of Long Island by myself.

Dale walked me through that. She did this methodically. She told me to sit in the driver's seat. She sat in the passenger seat. We put on our seat belts. I felt like a teenager taking a driving test. Off we went to Transitions of Long Island and back home. It was one of the most important drives for me and for Dale. It was for my dignity and control of a part of my life. For Dale it was a little piece of peace. She didn't have to come home right away from her job. She didn't have to chauffeur me back and forth to the park or barber shop or the supermarket. It was good for me and it was good for Dale.

Dale's elementary teaching skills made it easier for me. She planned the route precisely. Dale identified some landmarks before she rode with me in my car. She pointed out the landmarks, some of them I knew prior to my stroke. We drove north on Dogwood Avenue for about 1 ½ miles than a left on Nassau Boulevard. That was a piece of cake. That was where we shopped or the way I went to the North

Shore University Hospital. We made a right on Jericho Turnpike, than a quick left near Jonathan's restaurant on to Herrick Road. After Herrick Junior-Senior High School we made a left on to Manhasset Avenue and continued over both the Northern Parkway and the Long Island Expressway to Shelter Rock Road. At the junction of Shelter Rock Road and Northern Boulevard was a Lord and Taylor store. We made a right turn. Transitions of Long Island was about three blocks away on the right side. The building was painted Greek blue. This trip took about 35-45 minutes daily.

Rehabilitation at Transitions of Long Island

On February 25, 2002 I began my life again as a baby, infant, adolescent and an adult with the help of Transitions of Long Island. Transitions of Long Island placed a canopy over me and I suspect many of the other brain and stroke victims. I was free to see other people like me and I could laugh and cry and everyone would understand me. I didn't have to be embarrassed by my crying or fear. I always thought of Transitions of Long Island as a sheltered oasis from the first day but with a focused plan for me. For 15 months I received services at Transitions of Long Island from a multitude of professional women from speech pathologists to psychologists to secretaries to business administrators. They comforted, encouraged, guided and befriended me. Most of all they were very proficient, qualified and capable professionals. They helped me to improve my speech, my reading and my writing.

For the next 15 months the center of my day was the hour plus I spent in speech at Transitions of Long Island and my daily contacts with Peggy Kramer M.S, CCC-SLP and Deena Shein M.A. CCC-SLP. Ultimately, 90% of my time at Transitions of Long Island was spent with Peggy. She was my speech pathologist, my "psychologist" and my friend and that happened because she was a mature, bright, sensitive, funny, earthy, warm person. There was not one thing that she and I had not spoken about while I was at

Transitions of Long Island. Without these qualities I am sure that my gains would have been slower and more tedious. Throughout this book I will share vignettes and anecdotal stories about Peggy and myself as a means to show the scope and depth of my therapy and the manner in which Peggy's skills made my sessions with her meaningful and productive day in and day out. Our match was perfect because I needed a mature woman with real life experiences with marriage, kids, and knowledge about mature men and their dreams and fears and a task master.

Deena was a different person. There was about a 30 year difference in age between Peggy and Deena. Deena was young, with a beautiful face, with softness to her, and a proficient speech pathologist. Any man who has a son about 28-35 years old would love her for a daughter-in-law. She was a young competent speech pathologist and one who would grow in leaps and bounds in the future. Deena had wonderful human quantities, a warm smile, an easy laugh, empathy, strength of character and effortless conversational skills. I mentioned this because Peggy and Deena and all the other staff people see and deal with so much unhappiness, pain, misery and grief and yet they made my day productive and they humanized me, and they made me glad that I was alive.

I am sure that there were different courses that I had to relearn from first Deena and mostly from Peggy. One class focused on people with aphasia. Deena and Peggy understood that I had to overcome my aphasia in order to speak, read and write. Aphasia is an impairment of the ability to use or comprehend words. In other words I couldn't read one single sentence or one simple word. Throughout my stay at Transitions of Long Island all my work was woven together so that my speech was speech and an ability to use and comprehend words, reading was reading and an ability to use and comprehend words, and writing was writing and an ability to use and comprehend words. I know that my insurance company had problems in paying money to Transitions of Long Island for me for cognitive speech-language therapy services. I don't know and I don't want to know what the skill/service was. I knew that I was vexed by someone in the insurance company overruling the professionals who were giving me a chance to become "whole".

Throughout the first couple of months when you recoil from the shock as you gaze into an abyss of profound grief you must know that there will be some improvement in the condition of the your stroke victim. These gains may not be shown in tests. There may be anecdotal notes shared with you by the team or private therapist that works with your stroke victim. Listen and hear all the information that the team or private therapist shares with you. Pay attention to their interpretations of the different tests administered such as the Wechsler Adult Intelligence Scale-III (WAIS-III), selected subtests, Wechsler Adult Intelligence Scale-Revised Neuropsychological Instrument (WAIS-R-NI), selected subtests, Wechsler Memory Scale-III (WMS-III), selected subtests, Benton Visual Form Discrimination Tests, Finger Tapping Tests, Controlled Oral Word Association Test, Ruff Fluency Test, and Wisconsin Card Sorting Test (64 card, computerized version).

Please remember that these tests and others are formative diagnostic tools. They have real benefits for structuring programs for the patient. They are a lingua franca that allows the different specialties to talk with each other about the problems of patients. They provide direction for the staff and a way of assessing the growth of your stroke victim's progress for the insurance company. These tests are not sacrosanct but they do give professionals a better sense of direction for assisting their clients. Also they provide a means to make modifications rapidly to help their clients. One of the remarkable qualities of the staff, Peggy, Deena and the other therapists, and Debra Benson, Ph.D Clinical Neuropsychologist and Director, were their patience. They shared information and listened to my wife's anecdotal records about my performances and my thoughts on my deeds.

I never thought that I would have to take any academic tests ever again once I got my doctorate. Yet the tests that I took at <u>Transitions of Long Island</u> were the most important tests in my life. This chart shows you the skills that I had to learn or relearned by March 31, 2002 one month after I entered in to <u>Transitions of Long Island</u>. These were on a perfunctory level. You may ask your spouse's pathologist, coordinator or clinical director the names of the different tests used to evaluate his progress. These may not be formal tests. They may be just subtests from the CELF, MTDDA, BDAE and the Word Test. You might want to use this evaluation matrix as a way to see the frequency and amount of time spent of instruction on different skills and behaviors. It was clear that there were incremental gains some times and there were other times when there were no improvements at all or there was progress but they couldn't be seen in tests. The gains were so infinitesimal you needed to get anecdotal information from the staff.

Evaluation Finding

	Baseline data February 13, 2002	March 31, 2002
1.0 Auditory Disturbances		
1.1 recognize common words	18/18	
1.2 discriminate paired words	24/24	
1.3 recognize letters	21/26	
1.4 identify items named serially	6/6	
1.5 answered simple questions correctly	14/15	
1.6 followed oral directions	6/10	
1.7 asked yes/no questions related to a verbally presented paragraph	5/6	
1.8 repeat 2 and 3 digit numbers	Correct	Correct
1.9 repeat sentences	0/6	1/6
2.0 Visual and reading subtests		

2.1 match form to pictures	5/5	
2.2 match letters to pictures	20/20	
2.3 match words to pictures	32/32	
2.4 match printed to spoken words	32/32	
2.5 comprehended sentences based on yes/no format	14/15	
2.6 yes/no questions related to paragraph	6/8	
2.7 reading words	1/15	9/15
2.8 reading sentences	0/30	1/5
3.0 Speech and Language Disturbance		
3.1 imitated appropriate phonation, tongue movements, palatal movement and pharyngeal movements given a model by the clinician	Correct	
3.2 appropriate protrusion, retraction and lateral movement of his tongue	Correct	
3.3 repeat monosyllable words with difficulty noted towards the end of the list with blends (e.g. /sk/, /st/, /sch/, and /tr/).	26/32	30/32
3.4 repeat phrases	4/20	14/20
3.5 counting to 20 and reciting the days of the week	Correct	
3.6 completing sentences and answering simple questions related to using common objects	4/8	
3.7 asked to produce sentences given a stimulus word	0/6	Fair-good syntax
3.8 describing a picture	0/6	
3.9 name picture	4/20	14/20
4.0 Visuomotor and Writing Disturbances		
4.1 copy Greek	5/5	

4.2 copy numbers	20/20	
4.3 reproduce a drawing of a wheel with spokes	Correct	
4.4 reproduce letters	18/18	
4.5 writing letters to dictation	16/26	26/26
4.6 written spelling	2/10	9/10
4.7 oral spelling	0/10	4/10

From February 25 to March 31, 2002 Deena and Peggy taught me some compensatory strategies. My progress report said I was able to make active gains in the areas of confrontational naming, auditory comprehension at the sentence level, reading of words and phrases, and writing skills at the word level given dictation. My spontaneous speech showed significant improvement. I was able to repeat 2 and 3 digit numbers but none beyond, and 1out of 6 sentences, indicating continued difficulty with auditory recall. I was able to read 9 out of 15 reading words and 1 out of 5 reading sentences. Errors included marked slowness, inconsistent articulation, general slurring and substitution of words. I made gains when reading phrases and sentences. I showed improvement in repetition of monosyllabic words increasing from 26 out of 32 (2/13/02) to 30 out of 32 (3/31/02). I had difficulty with blends (e.g. /sk/, /st/, /skl/), however, there were improvements when a visual and/or verbal cue was provided. I continued to improve in repeating phrases from 4 out of 20 to 14 out of 20, however there was marked slowness and inconsistent articulation. My ability to produce sentences had significantly increased. I was able to produce a sentence when given a stimulus word with a fair to good syntax and 60% accuracy. I was able to name 14 out of 20 pictures, a significant increase from 4 out of 20 (2/13/02). My ability to write letters to dictation increased from 16 out of 26 to 26 out of 26, written spelling from 2 out of 10 to 9 out of 10, and oral spelling from 0 out of 10 to 4 out of 10. My spelling difficulties continued to be evident although I was able to use the compensatory strategy of writing the word that I was trying to say with greater accuracy.

These were words used for reports but they did mean that I was able to start relearning reading, writing, speaking and listening.

Yet, they also showed my marked slowness, inconsistent articulation, general slurring, and spelling difficulties and an inability for substitution of words. In other words I had very, very limited words that I could use. I was not able to spell words easily nor with any accuracy. I couldn't use synonyms for words that I couldn't say or spell. I had a very limited ability to form simple sentences and I slurred my speech. In the real world that meant that I was not able to speak with people that I didn't really know and I couldn't write my thoughts to those who I loved. Pretend that you are in your high school freshmen Spanish or French or Russian or Chinese or Arabic course 1. It is the first day of class. You are asked to speak to people who are fluent in each language. You also slurred. Nobody cared to listen to you because you made no sense. The words didn't make sense, the tenses made no sense, and the sentences made no sense. You slurred you speech. Add to that the frustration that you can't form your words in your mouth so that even though you knew a word you were not able to pronounce it and add to that, you had no other way to talk to the people in another language.

The classes/groups were made up of four to eight people plus Deena or Peggy or one of the other speech pathologists. Most of the rooms were small and sterile, few if any had pictures on the walls, the paint on the walls was bland, and yet there was great learning in these classes, momentous efforts by the men and women who wanted to be made "whole". Peggy, Deena and other therapists strained every day to help us to say a word or a simple sentence. Sometimes I saw their frustration not with the stroke victims but with themselves. It showed in the eyes of Deena, maybe because she was so young and her face was not wrinkled with experience. Yet in my one to one classes with Peggy initially I always saw the sadness in her face, from her mouth to her eyes, for me. She wanted me to get better and yet she was a professional who knew that there were other factors that she and I could not control. She and I tried hard to do all we could do and for that I will always be grateful for all her efforts on my behalf. As the days and weeks and months passed there were lots of smiles and laughter. At the end of my therapy with Peggy there were heartfelt conversations with pain and laughter.

Peggy Kramer, my Peggy Kramer

That first month, February 25 to March 31 2002, at Transitions of Long Island was very difficult and made the effort that I had put into my doctoral program kids play. From the first time I entered Transitions of Long Island the words Transitions of Long Island and Peggy Kramer were entwined. Throughout the entire time that I convalesced at Transitions of Long Island I saw Peggy, first as the Speech Coordinator for the program and my case manager and ultimately my speech teacher, "psychologist", confidant, and political collaborator against all that was wrong in the Bush administration. In other words Peggy knew all my thoughts about my fears about my stroke, my family and my professional goals. She helped me to become "whole" in ways that were important to me in my reading, writing, speaking and listening. It was a college friendship with the maturity of age and respect and intelligence and platonic love.

Deena, my Teacher

During most of this month I worked with Deena and Peggy but Deena spent more time with me. I was her client-patient in a real sense. Deena was about 27 years old and 5'2". She was blond and sweet. She had a winning smile and she was gentle. Most of the professional women, if not all, were warm and compassionate. They were well dressed, most often in casual pants or blouses and skirts and sneakers. There was a continuum of women from the twenties to the fifties. There was a sweet aroma that flowed in the air that made me aware that I needed to shower and groom myself to go to <u>Transitions of Long Island</u>. The smiles of these women were therapeutic and the ugliness of my life was dissipated. For the one and half hours I was in <u>Transitions of Long Island</u> I loved the smiles, aroma, makeup, lipstick, blouses, skirts and friendly concerns for me. All of these were part and parcel of Deena for the month of February 25 – March 31, 2002.

The classes were difficult for me. I had to print/write the name of the month, day, and date on a page by looking at the board in some of the classes. Sometimes I was not able to print/write them in time to start the lesson. During March I was asked to match pictures to phrases. There were many pictures and phrases. There was a face with a razor on one side of the page followed by a person drinking a cup of coffee, and a hand with a pen. On the other side of the page were the phrases-"drink coffee from it", "write with it", and "shave with it". I had to match the picture of the razor to the phrase that said "shave with it". It was somewhat difficult because I couldn't read the phrases well but I was able to match the phrases only because I could see the pictures and some of the letters.

After this exercise Deena had me match objects to actions. The process was similar to pictures and phrases but not quite. You see there were no pictures. The 20 objects were words such as razor, paintbrush, cup, dollar, flashlight, toothbrush and key. The actions were "unlock a door with it", "brush your teeth with it", "drink coffee from it", "buy things with it", "shine it in the dark", "paint with it", and "shave with it". It was more difficult because I couldn't read most of the objects and actions.

All of my sessions with Deena and later Peggy had some pragmatic/social conversations. From what I recall Deena started or ended our sessions with some question or a stimulus word and that allowed me to talk with her. Sometimes, in unrefined English, I told her about Erick's desire to go to Florida State University. I spoke to her so softly I couldn't hear myself. My speech voice had been altered by my stroke. It was difficult for me to find words for our conversations and look at her while I spoke to her. It wasn't because Deena wasn't beautiful, she was. It was that I couldn't look at anyone while speaking. I was not able to make eye contact regularly.

Deena suggested that I spend a little time on homework if possible. The homework turned out to be more arduous than anything I ever had in graduate school. I tried to work on my own but to no avail. It took one hour to show me that I needed help to learn the words in the area of objects and actions. It was an understatement. At about 7:00 p.m. Dale said she would help me with my homework. I tried to pronounce the words. I couldn't. Dale pronounced them and then I tried. Sometimes I got the word right, but most of the time I didn't. It took Dale and me four hours to finish my homework. Dale would enunciate the word and I would repeat it. Only I had to repeat the word over and over. I still wouldn't remember the word the next second. Dale said coffee. I said coffee. Dale said coffee. I said coffee. And then I tried again but I couldn't say coffee. Dale said cigarette. I said cigarette. Dale said cigarette. I said cigarette. And then I tried again but I couldn't say cigarette. Dale said eyeglasses. I said eyeglasses. Dale said eyeglasses. I said eyeglasses. And then I tried again but I couldn't say eyeglasses. I remember that I blurted out "fuck eyeglasses" not as a vulgar uncouth curse but as an instinctive character quality when faced with tremendous frustration. It was the end of the day and we both were spent emotionally and physically.

Although I knew that this was very difficult for Dale it took me many months to understand that it was not her job to work with me daily on the deficits in my speech or reading. She had a full time position as a teacher. She cleaned and cooked. I didn't begrudge her going to work probably because I went to Transitions of Long Island and I had work too. But it took a while for me to understand that it would not be beneficial for me or Dale to make her my speech teacher at home. On the other hand she did periodically listen to my reading and she did spell words to me when I couldn't sound out the words. She was my wife not my teacher and she was not a disinterested professional. On the contrary each time I said something or did something it had consequences for her twenty-four hours a day. That was the difference between my wife and my best friend at the time.

Dan, my Best Friend at <u>Transitions of Long Island</u>

The groups differed from class to class from day to day from person to person but there were a core of people who came together. One of them was Dan. Dan was about 60ish years old, silver hair, fair skin, and a gentle man, a good man. I think that Dan had a brain injury. He also had physical injuries. I think he had a broken jaw and broken legs or back. I think this sweet man had been hit in a car crash. I think but I don't know. We were like six month old children maybe with more salt and pepper hair. Yet Dan became my best friend in the whole world. We never spoke real words together. We tried. We tried to laugh together each day when we were in the same classes. It was wonderful to laugh together although we never knew what the details were that we were laughing about. We made faces. We looked around. We moaned. We smiled. There were the times that we both struggled to say a word any word. Seconds seem to be hours until the word formed in our mouths. Unfortunately, the word was not able to come out of the mouth. We were often left with sounds but no word, no recognized word during my first month at <u>Transitions of Long Island</u>. In frustration our eyes lowered, we slumped in our chairs or in Dan's case wheelchair and we cursed, not vulgar curses, just a drawing out of "shit". Usually, my daily hour at <u>Transitions of Long Island</u> ended and Dan and I hugged.

There were other people but I never remembered their names and for that I am sorry. They came in different races and religions, they were small and tall, they were thin and fat, they were women and men, they were poor and wealthy, they lacked family and they had families that loved and cared for them, they were part-time patients and full time patients –those who lived in the hospital. There were people who looked as if they were making strides, although how would I know in reality? I would only know about the people in my courses but I didn't know the difficulties they had and if I had I still would not know if they improved a little or a lot.

There were two women both about 30-40ish who I saw a couple of times a week for about one or two months. One had a brain injury as a result of a car accident. She was wheelchair bound. I remember that she had problems with words-she was more fluent than me in the first month of my stay at <u>Transitions of Long Island.</u> I thought that she was smart. In one of our classes I thought that she said that she was a public school teacher. She hungered for her three or four kids. One time the aide and the speech pathologist had to restrain her when she wanted to go home to her children. At that time she was not able to be coherent although anyone who heard her plaintive voice begging, as her cries and tears pierced the corridor, knew her pain. She must have seen herself as a woman alone on a ship in the northern Atlantic in February in the night with waves ripping over the ship, not able to see the sea and finding some comfort from the thought that all her pain would dissipate should she go into the Atlantic. Thank god for the medicine, aides and professional staff that helped her although these scenes still happened. Often in that month I remember that she wore a terrycloth bathrobe when she came to class. She had head surgery and her head was bandaged for weeks or months. After awhile she and I had different classes because we had different needs and abilities. However, I saw her a month or two or five after that and she was in the second floor corridor with her aide and some other staff people restraining her. Her dirty brownish blondish uncombed hair, framed a face, a classic Mediterranean face, perhaps of Portuguese origin, with tears from her eyes, nose and mouth. Her pain-even now-I must put my hands over my face and remember her trembling anguish yelling for her children, her scratched hands pulled over her hair, ripping her face, begging to be with them.

The other woman also fought with the aide and staff. She also wanted to go home to her children. She too had to be restrained, wailing, begging the staff to let her go home. She was frightened, humiliated and devastated. It wasn't because of any morale or spiritual misbehavior on her part. It was because strokes happen to good people also. Recently, in December, 2005 at a Christmas – Chanukah – holiday alumni party at Transitions of Long Island I saw her with her two or three children and her husband. Her children will never know how much their mother wanted to be with them. At the party I remembered the woman who was and I saw the "whole" person who is and the laughter of her children warmed the hearts of all the alumni in the room, the people who knew the agony that she went through.

There was a part time patient, a black woman, in one of my classes who also indicated that her essence was her children and cooking for them. As long as she could cook for them she was alive and she would deal with her handicap later. She too had aphasia. Her mouth started to form words but most of the time she struggled and stuttered and the words never came out. In our class she didn't appear to be embarrassed. She sat erect and made good eye contact. She tried and she tried as much as the other people in the class. Her husband was her problem and he muddied the waters because who knows. He was upset because she couldn't speak. It embarrassed him. She was sweet and the story was so sad.

Supporters

Throughout this period I had a support system that complemented the services I was given at Transitions of Long Island and more. Inadvertently but fortuitously, I had woven a support group made up by my wife, my son Jeff and daughter-in-law Anne, my friend Pierre, a health storeowner Fred, and teachers and administrators at the

Street Academy in New York City, Middletown City and Roosevelt School Districts. In different ways each and every person helped me with the nuances and subtleties needed to become a "whole" person, not a perfect person but a better Don Weinstein.

Neighborhood Helpers

It was about this time somewhere about March 10th that Dale and I went over to Fred's store-a health vitamin food fitness gym. I had known Fred for about eight years. Fred was about 40 years old, about 5'5 and about 130 lbs. and he had a cute face the kind of face that never ages. He had a MA in physical therapy. Before my stroke I worked out on the Nordic track and on the treadmill first running and then jogging and used some weights. I worked out for one Town of Hempstead half marathon and two or three small triathlons. In each of the triathlons I finished last but I enjoyed the thrill of the day. My wife (at that time she was my fiancée) and my sons watched me compete. My son Robert, when he was about 13 years old, helped me to finish the first triathlon race. I was so far off the pace of the rest of the people that Rob took his bike to find me and once he found me he paced me so that I finished the race. There was a police car that followed me also. The policeman cheered me on while he made sure that cars didn't hit me. My three sons and I played in three "Hoop It Up" Tournaments until I was 57 years old. I worked out for these at Fred's.

But Fred's was more than a jock and veggie hangout. In some ways it was a kind of New Hampshire country store without a stove and without a Robert Frost character. The veggie, vitamin, homeopathic and soy products made up about 500 square feet of the store. In March I tried to read the cereal labels and tried to pronounce the letters but to no avail. This section included the cash register counter area - a place to put all the vitamins until Fred totaled the bill. The rest of the 1200 square foot store was dominated by five treadmills, two Nordic tracks, two bikes, a nautilus, and free weights. It seemed to me that 85 percent of Fred clients were women most of whom were in the 40-60 a brackets. It was a gentle gym.

Fred liked to kibitz and talked about a variety of topics from politics and religion to features of the community and his customers. I had pushed Fred to write a physical fitness book. I nurtured him, suggested the format for the book and corrected and edited his writing. We finished this book maybe two or three months before my stroke. Unfortunately, Fred didn't follow some of my suggestions completely and it is still a manuscript. We had talked continuously about the 2000 election and the pros and cons of Gore and Bush and Cheney. Sometimes Lou, one of Fred's customers, played the game. We played and we laughed. I spent one hour one or two days a week at Fred's before my stroke.

I always thought that my strength was my ability to be facile with facts and ideas. These were residual benefits of my Latin American history doctorate and my background as an associate professor in education administration. In the past I would talk with Fred about Jewish, Christian and Muslim zealots or the nexus between Bush, oil, war and the destruction of the American dollar. Now I couldn't say two words together.

In the spring I spent 30 minutes three or four days a week going in to Fred's store and "speaking" with him. From the first day it was clear to me that Fred was overwhelmed or at the least shocked by the residual physical handicaps shown in my speech. Fred had told me that he couldn't understand my speech for two or three months but he listened to me and he said a couple of words to me and then I went home. I understood that I was either a pitiful soul, a wretched old man who had to talk to someone during the day or I was a person who didn't care how I got the time I needed to practice my speaking, reading and listening skills.

My time at Fred's also helped me to come to grips with my stroke. Every day that I was at Fred's I told another person

.nat I had a stroke and if they didn't understand me Fred told them. I talked and I talked and I talked and to me that was important. I also cried when I left the store but not for long. As I walked the two blocks home I tried to remember the words that I heard at Fred's and I tried to practice those words. I tried to pronounce them but I could not remember the letters much less the words. Most of the time I practiced one word if I was lucky. My time at Fred's supplemented my time at <u>Transitions of Long Island.</u> It gave me four more hours in speech skills and a better understanding of myself and other people. I was vulnerable but I didn't think that I needed to fear for my safety and I didn't believe that anyone would resort to witticisms or cruelty at my expense.

Fred's store was a gentle store and Fred was a kind man. Throughout my ordeal I saw Fred about three times a week from August 2002 to February 2005. Our conversations changed as I become more fluid. Most of our chats focused on politics and Bush's actions in Iraq. Fred would tell me that my speech was improving and by the end of September 2004 he said that he thought that my speech was 85 percent back to where I was before my stroke. By that time Fred decided that he didn't need to give me an advantage in our conversations. As a matter of fact he made sure that he spoke rapidly whenever he wanted to win a point. He knew that I couldn't talk quickly and I couldn't respond if he threw two thoughts to me at the same time. Once I knew his strategy I knew that this evangelist had a sense of humor, he was deceitful and played to win. But more than that Fred was a good person.

Tastes of Dignity and Humiliation

The gentleness found at Fred's store was not universal. It wasn't found at Key Food and it wasn't found at a neighborhood diner/restaurant. During the first week or two Dale made sure that everything that I needed was in the house especially lunch. I liked deli sliced Boar's Head low salt turkey, Chicken of the Sea solid white albacore tuna in water, oranges and twelve grain bread. After the first couple of weeks I needed to go to Key Food to by these items for lunch. Dale wasn't responsible to make sure that I had food for lunch. I could do that for myself. So I took a two block walk over to Key Food. It was good to feel the cold on my face as I walked the two blocks. And as I strolled I tried to think of the word "turkey". Once it came to me but in a second I forgot it. That was the conversation in my brain but unfortunately there was no dialogue with my speech.

Soon as I entered Key Food I froze I was anxious; would there be a line in the Deli counter, would I be able to say a couple of words, and would I be able to ask for turkey. The Deli woman was servicing another person. That allowed me to look around the deli area. There were advertisements one of which was for Boar's Head turkey. But I couldn't say it at that second. A couple of seconds later I was able to say turkey and I kept saying turkey over and over again. Than the deli woman asked me what I wanted. Those were the longest seconds because I couldn't remember the word "turkey". So I pointed to the advertisement. The woman asked me if I wanted Boar's Head or some or brand. I say "yes". She said Boar's Head and I said "yes". She asked me what kind and then she called out a litany of Boar's Head turkey products. I said "yes". She said some things. I said "yes". She asked me how much I wanted. She asked me if I wanted a half a pound or a pound. I said "yes". She asked me if I wanted a pound. I say "yes". She cut the turkey, weighed, packaged it, put the price on it and gave it to me and wished me a good day. As I walked out of Key Food I heaved a sigh. That sigh was more important than any sigh I felt after any BA, MA, or Ph.D. course. That sigh was more important than any sigh I felt after a teacher evaluation, administrative evaluation or college evaluation. That sigh indicated that I was able to feed myself. The Deli counter woman was wonderful. She was considerate and helpful. I never knew whether she understood intuitively the depth of my handicaps. But that didn't make any difference to me. What was unique was that she made me feel comfortable and treated me with dignity at a time when myself respect was shaky.

In juxtaposition to the deli counter woman there was a deli counter man and a waitress who were inconsiderate at best and vicious at worst although the possibility was that they were just ignorant. Every couple of days I took a walk to Key Food to buy a pound of low sodium Boar's Head turkey for lunch. That would hold me for two or three days. Periodically, the deli counter woman was not there and her replacement was the deli counter man. If deli counter woman was sensitive and accommodating deli counter man was abrupt and discourteous. He made me feel that I was an affront to him that I was grotesque. These feeling were in his speech in his inflections and intonations.

Hemoglobin Brain Man Versus Deli Counterman

I was a three part person; a brain, a mouth with a tongue and a torso with arms and legs. But the brain was the key. There was Hemoglobin Brain man, the master of the brain. Most of the time he takes surfboard rides in the blood vessels that brings oxygen and nutrients to the brain. Once in awhile he was not able to ride the waves in the blood vessel. There were some jams and he crashed and burned. Hemoglobin Brain man did not get the blood and oxygen I needed for my brain. Parts of my brain couldn't work and the parts of the body they control couldn't work either. Because Hemoglobin Brain man couldn't function or couldn't function well I couldn't speak, read, write and hear at all or with difficulty. Somewhere in my brain, Hemoglobin Brain man must have had a laugh at my expense groping for sounds and words. I was a puppet controlled by Hemoglobin Brain man. I sounded like a smashed drunk groping for sounds. Sometimes I laughed at myself and I scoffed at the people who thought I was an idiot but I despised this common bland round headed deli counter man.

There was a boorish coarseness to him. Yet, I never knew whether he was crude and vicious, just a Cossack, in his white frock or just stupid unable to get the slightest hints of my handicaps. The dialogue with deli counter man went something like this:

Deli Counter Man – Who's next? (I was the first person on line)
Yea? (No smile) What do you want? Come on what to you want? (I wasn't sure that I could say "me" or "yes" much less what I wanted.)
Me –Turkey.(I used up all my energy when I blurted out my order)
Deli Counter Man – What kind of turkey do you want? Come on I don't know what you want. Tell me what you want? (I didn't hear all his words and I had to focus on one question at a time.)
Me – I point to the flyer next to counter. (Thank God for the gray flannel suites in advertisements and the men and women who work on Madison Avenue throughout the country.)
Deli Counter Man – Boar's Head all right?
Me – Yes. (I wasn't sure whether the word that he said was Boar's Head.)
Deli Counter Man – What kind of Boar's Head? What do you want? Come on I'm waiting? (I felt livid because he pushed me for no reason; he was just malicious and I wished my professorial self would cut him with my sharp tongue; I couldn't and I didn't.)
Me – I look at the ad pensively for a couple of seconds. (I couldn't read the ad but it made me a little calmer as I looked at the ad.)
Deli Counter Man – You want (whatever he said).
Me – Yea. (You contemptible nauseating bastard)
Deli Counter Man – OK what do you want?
Me – I look pensively.
Deli Counter Man- Did you say a pound?
Me – Yea.

This exchange took a minute or so but it was excruciatingly painful and humiliating. After a second or two, Deli Counter Man knew or sensed that I had a speech handicap but he continued to push me to answer his queries quickly.

As more people lined up for service from Deli Counter Man he became more surly and it seemed to me as if he was trying to play to the other customers at my expense; the rolling eyes and looking back and forth to the other people.

Now I go to Key Food periodically to buy some odds and ends including turkey from Deli Counter Man. I know that he is perplexed by my speech and manner. After all I appear to be one of the "normal" people. How sad for me that I now deal with him as an inept person inadequate and hopeless.

My Wife and the Waitress

What I wrote was excruciatingly painful for Dale. Dale saw the anger that flooded these pages the rage that consumed me. Yet, there was no doubt that Dale did all that she could do and more and she loved me in tangible ways. These pages were testimony of that and her needs and fears also although they were not depicted in such raw descriptions. Dale has her own way to help other wives or girlfriends of stroke victims. If it wasn't for Dale I would not have improved as quickly as I had. In every way in every manner I loved Dale. I was only able to paint pictures that were stored in my brain.

Early March 2002 a couple of weeks after my hospitalization Dale and I went out for breakfast in a neighborhood diner/restaurant, one that we ate regularly on Saturdays and Sundays for 10 years. Our regular waitress, who was about 50, and chatty, came over to find out why we hadn't been in. Dale told her. The waitress gasped and then she asked for our orders. Dale ordered for both of us. I hadn't asked her to do that. Dale thought it would save me from any embarrassment. She probably was right. But I wanted to try. She took that away from me but she was probably right. A couple of weeks later we went back to the restaurant for breakfast again. We were seated. Then I looked around and I saw a table with four couples all about sixty to seventy years old. I had seen them regularly before but I never paid any attention to them. They were part of the diner/restaurant furniture every weekend. Now I had an intuitive feeling. I didn't see one of the men talking or ordering his food. His wife was ordering his breakfast. Periodically, he looked at the other people at his table. He just ate. He was not part of the conversations. I realized that he had a stroke. I never really found out if he had a stroke or brain injury but it didn't manner at all. I saw what I saw.

At that precise moment the waitress came over to take our order. Dale gave her order. Then the waitress instinctively looked at me. She was going to take my order. I had planned to give my order. At <u>Transitions of Long Island</u> I learned to read the word and sound out the word "egg". Sometimes I got it right. From the time that Dale and I drove to the restaurant from our house I focused on the word "egg" so I could order my food by myself. It took ten minutes to get to the restaurant. By the time we got there I couldn't guarantee to myself that I could say the word "egg". I started to give my order. I stuttered once or twice as I tried to say the word "egg". In less than a nanosecond the waitress looked at Dale for my order and didn't look at me for any conformation. This waitress, who knew me for years, couldn't or wouldn't allow me to have a couple of seconds or minutes to speak the word "egg". In the course of her job would it have been so terrible if she allowed me the time I needed to say "egg"? I knew this woman for years and she couldn't let me try to say "egg". And would it have been so terrible if Dale had said to the waitress give Don a couple of seconds to give his order to you? In the end I'm sure that I couldn't have done it but would it have caused any problems if I were allowed to try? Dale didn't want to shake up people. She thought her subtleness would help. She ordered both breakfasts as we held hands and we "talked" about Alison and Jessica. But there were buts lots of buts otherwise I would die and one of those buts was the word 'egg".

Reading as a Nursery Student

My speech was important to me, my ability to read was essential to me and my ability to write was vital to me. There was a symbiotic relationship between all three and therefore I needed to try to read as a first step to my recovery. That meant that I needed to learn to read again and that meant that I needed to go to the West Hempstead library to get some books. Dale and I took a drive over to the library. Dale had been a nursery school teacher when we met. She joined the public school system as an elementary school teacher and she had been responsible for elementary science since she got her job. Dale and I walked over to the nursery books in the library. There were three kids, somewhere between 3 to 4 years old, sitting on the floor talking and reading together. I looked for a book, one that I could read. Unfortunately, there weren't any. Dale picked out a book, one that had two to three sentences on a page. I don't remember the title but the gist of the book was "I said it was a horse" and each page added words. That night I tried to read the words and sentences but to no avail. I tried to say "I" aloud. Sometimes I got the word "I" right. Oftentimes I didn't. But by the time we went to bed I got the word "I" in some part of my mind. It was difficult for me to say "said" aloud. It took me about a month or so to finish that little nursery book and it took so much energy to read it. It took a lot out of Dale also.

At the same time Dale got some of her colleagues to give me some lists of words used by nursery to first graders. There were lists of "it" words – bit, fit, hit, pit; and lists of "at" words – bat, cat, fat, and hat. After we ate Dale listened to me as I tried to sound out the words and repeat the words again. It was tedious for me and Dale. She talked about her work day and how difficult it was for her to go through the two to four hours of my "homework". I was trying to get my life back and I was not sensitive about her physical and emotional needs. Dale should have been frazzled. She should have been upset because she didn't have a second to herself. It was like a new mother with a frustrated and resentful 63 year old husband. At the same time my priority was my life. In about a week I came to the conclusion that I could only count on myself to get better and the truth be known, that was true. That was not because Dale or Jeff didn't care or love me. They did. It just meant that I needed to put more energy in to myself. My thoughts were best said in the Kingston Trio song The Reverend Mr. Black. The chorus says "I gotta walk that lonesome valley. I got to walk it by myself. Oh nobody else can walk it for me. I got to walk it by myself".

Dale loved me in significant ways; the ways that Golde sings to Tevye in Fiddler on the Roof. There were so many things that Dale did for me. Dale helped me with my pills; she put my pills in those weekly boxes and I had two boxes, one for the morning pills and one for the night pills. She made sure that my pills were always ready from the pharmacy. She cooked our suppers from Monday to Thursday and she was superb. Her salmon dishes and shrimp and pasta dishes were fabulous. We had a glass of merlot to wash down the meals. There was fresh grain bread with extra virgin olive oil. Dale cleaned the table and put the dishes in the washer every day. She washed our clothes weekly. Dale periodically helped me with my speech, reading and writing but not regularly and never as a tutor. And yet in my gut at that time I thought it was more important for me to have Dale involved in my 'homework" than pills, cooking, and washing.

Stroke Victim, Blended Family and Holidays

Dale and I tried to forge a secular Jewish-Lutheran blended family together as only an American New Yorker can do. Periodically, Dale came with me to shul (synagogue) for Rosh Hashanah and Yom Kippur. Sometimes Jeff, Anne, Alison, Jessica, Robert and Erick joined us in shul. I went with Dale to church on Christmas Eve two or three times. In some fashion we succeeded and in others we failed.

Pesach and Pickle Day

One of the best times were the holidays especially Pesach, Passover. We made pre Pesach a ritual as only non religious Jews and Christians can. We knew the cultural, religious and historical events of Judaism. We knew about the Israeli-Palestinian conflicts and death and the outburst of Anti-Semitism periodically in the United States, Europe and Argentina. Two and a half weeks before Passover on March 17, a Sunday, Jeff, Anne, Alison, Jessica, Erick, Mark, Dana, Dale and I met on the Lower East Side of Manhattan. We met on Grand Avenue and Delancey Street and walked over to Gus's pickles, a landmark. The smell of the horse radish, lines of customers, and the chatter of people who came from the suburbs spells Pesach to me.

We waited on line by Gus's pickle store, with fifty or more people in a street that was no wider than six or seven feet and talked to one another about the little and big things, the stuff that makes blended families blended. How were Alison and Jessica? Was Jessica feeling better from her heart surgery? How was Robert? Were Mark and Dana concerned about the pregnancy? And Anne and Jeff asked Dale about me and asked me about me also. There was gossip about who was coming to Pesach. Would Ariena come because she was in her freshman year in the University of Pennsylvania? Would Carlton and his children come? After all, he was a terrific person and his kids added warmth to the Seder and it made my oldest and warmest female cousin Dorothy happy to see her grandchildren around her at Pesach. Smell all of those half sour, full sour, and hot spicy pickles, garlicky tomatoes, sweet red peppers, olives, marinated mushrooms and sauerkraut. Make sure that you get a whiff of fresh horse radish, the odor which you can smell half a block away.

Most of the people on line talked about the powerful horse radish as did we but I was not me in my usual way. I was not glib. I did not interject information about the history of the Lower East Side and the Jewish legacies all around us such at the First Romanian American Synagogue, at 89

Rivington Street, one block north of Delancey Street between Ludlow and Orchard Streets and the unions that put up the apartment building on Grand Avenue. I did not talk about the Yiddish theaters that my parents and grandparents, Poppa and Bubba, took my aunt and me when I was 5 or 6 years old. I did not talk about the Henry Street Settlement House. I did not talk about my Bar Mitzvah in Pollack's catering restaurant in June, 1951. I did not talk about the schools in the Lower East Side that I worked in as a recreation leader when I first married.

I did smile when someone on line said something funny most probably about their grown up children, something about enjoying their newly empty nest when their adult child decided to move back in. I smiled when I said "yes" to somebody's question and it was clear to me that no one knew that I had a limited vocabulary. There were jokes about the double parking in the street and the traffic cops that allowed it to happen and the need to go back to the roots of one's childhood memories. I did smile when Dale, Anne and Jeff were laughing. I smiled when I walked over to a store a couple of stores away to buy Poland Spring water and came back with the water that I bought to no one's surprise. I was able to say some words, point out what I wanted, and made some gestures, paid with a five dollar bill, and got the change. Consequently, I was part of the real world again as long as I did not take more time than the store owner or worker wanted to give me.

I smiled once I knew that Dale, Anne, Jeff, Alison and Jessica had a great time and my childhood memories and knowledge really would not add or decrease the laughter. I was able to sit back and enjoy the fresh air of the Lower East Side, the smells of Grand Avenue and Essex Street, and the laughter of the people that I loved and myself. I smiled as Dale, Anne and Jeff told the men in Gus's what they wanted and the way Dale, Anne, Jeff, and Alison ate their pickles and Jessica was given a taste of the water from a pickle. Dale and I bought a couple of pints of red and white fresh ground horse radish for the Seder. Then Anne and Jeff put all their quarts of pickles and tomatoes into their car. They had made a run for Anne's parents and sisters and brother-in-laws. Everyone knew the magic of Gus's pickles for Pesach. Dale and I put all the pickles, tomatoes, sauerkraut and fresh horse radish into my car. This would have been enough for me to be happy and thankful if I was well. Can you imagine the excitement? One month after my stroke I was part of my family, with my granddaughters in sight, in the midst of childhood memories sweetened by the lives I nurtured and loved.

But there was more. There was Katz's Deli, the oldest deli in New York City, on 205 East Houston Street, with the best pastrami and corn beef sandwiches, pickles, coleslaw, hotdogs and French fries washed down with a Dr. Brown's Cel-ray soda or two. Katz's was a slow meandering thirty minute walk from Gus's via Orchard Street and the multitude of men's wear, leather, handbags, children's clothing, fabrics, luggage, electronics, computer and umbrella stores. From Delancey Street to Houston Street were reminiscences of pushcarts and peddlers, the memories of my childhood. On Sundays Orchard Street was closed to cars. It was made into a pedestrian street mall. Throughout this stroll I looked at the facades on the stores and tried to say the words or at least the letters. Once in awhile I said "no" to one of the hawkers of clothing or baggage. I always said "thanks" when one of the peddlers asked me to touch a garment or toys or wallets. This was a street of unpretentious people. It felt wonderful on Orchard Street. I was able to walk leisurely and glance at the stores and people walking on the street. My senses were alert. There was the fresh wind on my face. There were the aromas of roasted peanuts and hotdogs and the sounds of people laughing and talking. I glimpsed at the diversity of buildings, restaurants, and stores. My family didn't have any concerns about my dawdling and I didn't need to reassure them that I was safe and happy. I was just taking a walk. Sometimes Dale and I walked together. Other times I walked with Jeff and Anne. It was fantastic when Alison and I sauntered on Orchard Street. She and I looked for sunglasses for her. She asked me about the glasses she put on and she allowed me to answer her question with a "yes" or a gesture of thumb up. Life was good.

At Katz's we met Mark and Dana for lunch. It was a sumptuous and cheerful meal. Remember, this was the place where Meg Ryan demonstrated her orgasmic skills in <u>When Harry Met Sally</u>. The place was crammed the side for waiter service was jam-packed. The others, Jeff, Dale, Anne, Alison, Mark and Dana, were a little upset because it would take 10 to 15 minutes to get a table at this time of the day. As they strategized I found one of the managers and asked him in words and gestures for a table for nine including Jessica. He took me to the end of the deli and made a right and there were large tables meant to fit 15 to 20 people. I found my family group. They were mesmerized, they doubled up laughing. They could not believe that I was able to be so useful and creative. I got us a table. Dale told me when I wrote this chapter that they laughed because it was clear the Freddie Kruger Weinstein was back and fit. Our meal was relaxing, the company was congenial, and I saw my granddaughters again in a lovely setting, the linkage of my past, my present and all of my futures.

After we ate at Katz's we took a stroll over to Yonah Schimmel's for knishes, the best knishes because they were baked not fried and they were a legacy of a rabbi from Romania, my grandfather's country of origin. As we strolled the two blocks to Yonah Schimmel's I walked with Mark and Dana separate from the rest of the group. Once again I tried to speak but I don't remember if my speech made any sense. What I do remember was that Mark and Dana kept looking at each other after I said something or other. I guessed that I didn't make any sense to them. Look, I don't know what went on in my brain. I surely didn't know what was in their minds. It was clear that I couldn't communicate in any meaningful way. But in that moment I knew that I did the right thing when I decided to go to <u>Transitions of Long Island</u>.

Pre Pesach and the Merry Maids

All of this was a prelude to Pesach on March 28. I say March 28 because Dale and I made the Seder on the second night of Pesach. This allowed all of our guests the luxury of spending time with other family members and friends on the first night of Passover. Also it gave us one more day to clean the house. It would have been difficult for us if we didn't hire the Merry Maids. They sent a swat team of three women to clean the kitchen, dining room, living room, three bathrooms and four bedrooms.

When they finished their work I had to write them a check. I was confused. I couldn't understand the bill in words or numbers. It took five minutes or so for the woman in charge of the team to understand that I needed help. She wrote the number $325.79 or so. That was a number but I couldn't understand the words. I didn't know have to pronounce that number. I tried but I just couldn't. Then I tried to write the check. That was a nightmare. It seemed that these women only spoke Spanish. I didn't speak Spanish. Finally, one of the women spelled out the number for me on a white sheet of paper. That was how I was able to write that check. It was mortifying, but it passed. More importantly, I paid the Merry Maids with a check in my own handwriting. These women didn't want to degrade me. They were nice women. They just wanted a check. As the days passed in to weeks, months and years there would be others who took delight in trying to degrade me but not at that time and place.

The Seder

Our Pesach was superb. The people were genuinely nice. They were interested in each other. They were lively. There was a blend of granddaughters, twenties to forties, and the plus fifties. Our group consisted of Jews, Christians, agonistics, and atheists. But they had a common purpose to spend time with family and friends. There was Anne, Jeff, Alison and Jessica. There was Cousin Bernie and Connie.

My mother and father loved Bernie from the time he was a baby. Connie was terrific. She was warm, honest, and nice. She had an earthly quality. Bernie's son Seth was warm also and charming. Dorothy was Bernie's sister and the oldest living member of my father's side of my family. I had a crush on Dorothy when I was in high school and college. I have always thought of her as an Aunt Mame person. She and Bernie were the historians in the family. There was Carlton. He was the ex son-in-law of Dorothy and he had to be one of the most extraordinary people I have met. He made sure that his grownup children spent an evening with their grandmother and their extended family. Dorothy's grandchildren were Adrian, Vanessa, Hunter and Scarlett. Unfortunately, there were a number of young adults who were not able to participate in this Seder. Most of them were in college and it was nearing test time.

Dale prepared a great Seder dinner for approximately 25 family members and friends. She bought chopped liver as an appetizer. There were matzos, sodas, wines and liquors. People ate chopped liver and matzo and drank. They mingled got the feel of each other and renewed their friendships. The oldest wanted to make sure that the youngest were healthy and flourishing and that those in school were thriving. Young adults chatted about college and their professions and travels. Dale, Anne and Connie wanted to hear the thought of one of the young adults who acted with Robert Redford. Jeff and Bernie spoke one-to-one. Dorothy, Seth and Carlton talked. But the truth was that the conversations flowed as people chatted with other people. Dale's Seder included gefilte fish with horseradish, chicken soup with matzo balls, a twenty pound turkey, vegetable, potatoes, and pickles. There was soda and Malaga and Concord wines and merlots. The merlots were for the Christians, agnostics and atheists. There was coffee and kosher cake and candies, especially the chocolate covered matzos, for Pesach.

Dale and I greeted all our guests at the door but I didn't know whether they knew that I had had a stroke. We hugged and I guess I said something but I don't know what and I don't remember what the others said except Dorothy. She told me that she had a stroke too and she was certain that I would be able to come back to my old self. After that I melded in with one group of relatives after another. I had nothing to offer to the conversations after the first couple of seconds. I listened and I laughed and I was very happy to have had all these people to our Seder. Dale and I made the best decision when we decided to have the Seder in our home. For the past 15 years we had Seders at our home. It was important to continue that tradition at least for the foreseeable future.

One of the sweetest sights happened immediately. As people ate their appetizers I played with Alison and Jessica in "their" bedroom. We colored and they talked, especially Alison. They chatter with each other. They lay on the floor and colored and negotiated for different crayolas. They talked continuously. I loved their voices when they made the sounds of "grandpa". I thought that that would be my lot for the rest of my days sitting and talking with my granddaughters while adults sat in the other rooms laughing, telling jokes, and providing insights about the problems with Bush and Cheney. I was reconciled to this fate almost at once, a fate that was sad in some ways. After about forty minutes or so Alison joined the other ladies. Jessica took my hand and walked me though the house. She looked at the pictures on our walls and the photos of her and the rest of the family. Jessica asked me questions about some of the people in the photos. She smiled that beautiful wide smile often as she walked with me hand in hand from room to room not caring whether my speech was fluent or not. She just wanted to walk and talk with her grandpa, me. Quickly, I knew that I wanted this for me forever, talking, walking, coloring and singing with my granddaughters, Alison and Jessica. How strange was divine intervention or providence? My stroke helped me to understand that my time with Alison and Jessica was more important than the witticisms of politics.

Prior to my stroke before the actual Seder I thanked all my guests for honoring us with their presence. I told them the joys that happened to me from the previous Pesach to the present Pesach. Then each member of my extended family told us some positive event for them over the past year. All of us heard their thoughts. Although this was a tradition in my home it was an abridged version of my childhood memories. I lived with my grandparents and parents and my uncles and aunt in a three bedroom apartment in East New York. My grandfather conducted the Pesach services. The service was in Hebrew. The Four Questions were read by me. I had to read them in Hebrew, Yiddish and English. My bubba, mother and aunts cooked for hours maybe for days for Pesach. I remembered the services when my poppa read in Hebrew the answers for the Four Questions and I and all the men read along with him. Sometimes the Seder ended at 1:00A.M when everyone sang in a robust voice HAD GADYA.

I tell you this so that you could understand the anguish when I knew that I had to turn over the Seder to Jeff and Bernie. The distress was minimal once the time came. Dale was the mistress of the house. She talked to everybody. She looked out for everyone-food, drinks. She prepared the table and the Seder plate with Egg, Shank Bone, Bitter Herbs and Heroseth. It was her vivacious personality that helped others to feel more comfortable. I tried to tell my extended family that I was happy for their appearance at this Seder and that Jeff and Bernie would conduct the services.

I was not sure they got all my words but they got the essence of my thoughts. I remember that I had four thoughts at that time. First, I was glad that all these people came to the Seder and that they didn't make me feel that I was an 800 pound gorilla in their midst. Second, I didn't want Jeff to feel uncomfortable for me. He should have his own Seder if I couldn't in the future. Third, I wanted Jeff and Bernie to make sure that all the people were comfortable. As a matter of fact they were terrific, they got a couple of laughs and they were a good duet. Last, I was glad for the help given to me by Deena and Peggy. I heard and felt my progress. I heard it through the comments of my family and the words in the Passover Haggadah read by my extended family.

But the most cherished moment of the Seder for me was when Anne, holding Jessica, and Alison sang the Four Questions so softly, so sweetly, and so tenderly. All of the people hung on each sound. This was the gift of life for me, my Jeff's wife singing with my granddaughters seated next to me. Stroke or no stroke life was good to me at that Seder and probably I should remember that feeling for the rest of my life; that love, that respect and that honor.

Conclusion

It was unambiguous from the first second that I came home. Dale, Jeff and Anne wanted to make my life productive at once. No isolation, loneliness and helplessness for me. As a result within one month they helped me to structure daily "work" activities. I "talked" with Pierre every morning at 7:10 a.m. and Fred somewhere between 1:30-4:00 p.m. I made my lunch, drove to and from Transitions of Long Island. I "spoke" to secretaries and guards at Transitions of Long Island, and attended my classes with Deena or Peggy. I inputted data to my time-on-task program so that teachers in the Maple Hill Elementary School in Middletown, New York would know the instructional time spent on English and math daily. I worked on my homework, "talked" with Dale in the evening and watched television. I went to my doctors by myself. Once a month I went to North Shore University Hospital to take blood tests. Every Friday night we went for dinner at a neighbor Italian restaurant and every Saturday morning Dale and I went for breakfast. There was the joy of going to the Lower East Side with my family and especially my granddaughters Alison and Jessica. There was the human warmth that the Passover Seder held for me-my past, present and future.

Inextricably intertwined was my clash between my full daily life and my infantile behavior. There was my inability to make consistent eye contact. My speech was soft and tenuous. I was powerless to talk with two people at the same time or to have one person talk to me quickly. I didn't foresee the pain that my youngest son, Erick experienced. He was overwhelmed by my nakedness. Sometimes I saw pity from acquaintances and strangers. I wanted to tell them not to feel sorry for me. I had a better life than I thought possible. I was a real person, with family to love, and dreams to dream. I couldn't. But I tried.

Checklists

Victim needs to:
1. Make sure that they continue to try to speak or use gestures to convey their thoughts every time they get a chance.

2. Require people, such as doctors, clerks, and waitresses to give them the time to say whatever they need to say with dignity and to decide when they need help to express themselves.

3. Chat with family members during breakfast, lunch, and dinner and listen to the discussions also.

4. Get a notepad and write down any words that you want to know. If you can write the word great if not ask someone to help you to write out the word and pronounce it, probably two to five times.

5. Make sure that they sit down at the table with all other adults in any gathering and allow the natural conversations to go on.

6. Listen to television and radio. They need to try to say a word or two that they just heard.

Family members need to:

1. Please relax; that means some television, talk about themselves or other family members or friends or acquaintances or news items, drink a glass of wine or beer, talk on the telephone, and just relax.
2. Please make sure that you treat your spouse as a mature person with respect and dignity.

3. Please don't push your stroke victim hard because you are embarrassed by his impairments. The truth is that you need to make it clear to the world that you want the rest   of the world to treat your spouse/significant other with respect. The time is so insignificant- thirty second, doesn't your spouse deserved thirty seconds?

4. Please stop correcting your husband/wife's speech. It is reasonable to correct a couple of words once in a while, which means it is acceptable if your spouse says it is acceptable. You are not their speech pathologist. Talk with his/her speech pathologist to see what the speech pathologist wants you to do.

Chapter 3: April 2002-July 2002 My Unfolding Passage on the Continuum from Stroke Victim to Stroke Survivor

Review

This chapter is the first of two chapters, the other is Chapter 4 that point out my progression from stroke victim and the steps needed to become a functional person, to stroke survivor. In order to get both the big picture and details about my interaction with people, agencies and institutions, I need to share the results of a neuropsychological report about me written in June 28, 2002 by the professionals at <u>Transitions of Long Island</u>.

This report detailed information about my disabilities and offered a realistic perspective of my limitations by the end of June. It afforded a framework with which to view my interactions with my loved ones and the people in agencies and institutions that were my clients. I suspect that a researcher could use my actual life (or anyone else's) performances and the constraints reported on June 28 and set a baseline and evaluate my growth and place that growth in a continuum of behaviors. But it isn't necessary. Just look at the three major subject matters in this chapter their subtleties and nuances and form your own conclusions as you read about my:
- ◊ medical issues, my neuropsychological report, my daily work at <u>Transitions of Long Island</u>, changes in my medication, my physical exercise routine and my psychological therapy.
- ◊ consultancy, making presentations, working with educators and proofing work.
- ◊ family and my extended family.

Neuropsychological Report

When I wrote this chapter three years after "graduating" from <u>Transitions of Long Island</u> it was the first time I actually read the Neuropsychological Evaluation Report about me written on June 28, 2002 eleven days after my 64th birthday. It was painful to read even after those three years. I put my hands over my head as I read the report with both detachment and horror. I had nightmares for days. My wife said there were low prolonged moans in my sleep and I thrashed my arms and legs. Had I read this report and understood the jargon in the report in June 2002 it would have devastated me and my family but the report was solely for the use of the professionals at <u>Transitions of Long Island</u> and the insurance company. I thought that I had made gains especially from April to June. In retrospect, I had more problems than I thought once I read the report. The fact that I didn't interpret the report in June 28th meant that I didn't have to back myself into a self fulfilling prophesy because of the report.

When I read the report I was struck by my lack of knowledge of neuropsychological language, a gobbledygook of words that made no sense to me such as "remarkable" as in "remarkable for multiple…" or "There his aphasia improved markedly…" and "premorbid". It didn't comfort me to read the terminology in the report as "relative strength" when I didn't know the definition of "relative strength" and how this compared to "Superior range", "Low Average range", "with healthy limits", "relatively low performance", "Impaired range", "borderline range" and "expressive aphasia" and the comment that my "relatively strong performance on the Matrix Reasoning Test can be attributed to the fact that he was not required to give a rapid response."

This evaluation showed me that four months after I enrolled in <u>Transitions of Long Island</u> I had difficulties in language, processing speed, attention, some aspects of memory, visuospatial functioning and problem-solving. The evaluator estimated my cognitive functioning prior to my stroke in the "Superior" range. These tests demonstrated scattered ability from one domain to another and within each domain. As I waded through the jargon, standard scores and percentiles I felt like a knight-errant looking for a virgin in a blues club on Bleecher Street on a summer's evening. I knew what I was looking for but how would I tell by looking alone. How could I tell whether the cute brunette was a virgin or the cute blonde? There were six domains in the evaluation and approximately 25 tests and subtests and how would I know the significance of each test and subtest? I knew the big picture from the summary of the evaluation but I didn't know what limitations were on the tests and the way the scores were interpreted. Without these I would be foolish to try to reinterpret these tests even if I could and I couldn't and on June 28th I had language, speech and writing handicaps.

This evaluation was for the purpose of assessing my present level of cognitive functioning. Gross receptive language appeared intact however I had significant word finding difficulties and minor dysfluency. On one occasion, when I experienced the answer on "the tip of his tongue" I spontaneously began to write the answers to questions. It indicated that my written language was not as impaired as my spoken language. My speech was observed to be somewhat slow and low in volume.

I don't know whether I actually thought about what I would read once I was able to read proficiently. I didn't know whether I would read and interpret the classics from the Torah to Shakespeare to Stein and everything in between or whether I would read the light paperback books shown in the New York Times, the books that I read prior to my stroke at night to get to sleep or to sleep on the beach. But what I did know was that I would not take any more of my time, so precious was time, to read the Tweedledee and Tweedledum articles in educational journals, res ipsa loquitor (the things speaks for itself).

I was surprised at myself when I decided to read my evaluation in earnest. I didn't know whether it was another Tweedledee and Tweedledum report, another boilerplate report filled with my data. It turned out that this was a sober description of my intellectual, arousal and attention, language, memory, visual-spatial and frontal lobe functioning. After I read the details the only thing I could think about was that if this type of report was used for sex Adam and Eve probably would have had to look at lots of pretty flowers, beautiful sunsets, and striking mountains because they wouldn't understand the jargon of sex in the report and the natural act of sex would be lost on them.

I didn't know what these tests and percentile scores meant in truth. Did a 37th percentile score mean that I was below average, average, high average, or superior in the specific test, and did I have to just add or subtract to come to a conclusion or were there formulas and were these formulas usable and practical for me and you? There were lots of tests and subtests and tremendous percentile ranges from one test to another test and between domains. I didn't know how to calculate all of these percentiles and come to specific conclusions. Was there a weight to each test and subtest and each percentile? Ultimately, it was clear to me that I needed to have Peggy interpret all these data for me and I didn't at that time at least that was my recollection maybe. You get a glimpse of the vast scope of the test assessment program just for one domain.

Tests showed that I had major problems in intellectual functioning. The test assessed my verbal comprehension at the 53rd percentile, working memory at the 1st percentile, information at the 75th percentile, and Letter Number Sequencing at the 1st percentile. My verbal comprehension was scored at the 37th percentile and Similarities was scored at the 50th percentile. They were at the "average" range. But Arithmetic was scored at the 9th percentile, and Digit Span at the 5th percentile. They were "relatively low". On the Matrix Reasoning Test I scored at the 63rd percentile, Picture Completion Test at the 2nd percentile and Block Design at the 37th percentile, an "average" range. Digit Symbol Coding was scored at the 25th percentile, in the "low Average" range.

There was a great deal that I didn't know about my brain prior to my stroke and I surely didn't know much about the jargon related to the brain and tests, score percentiles, and interpretation of tests. You should make sure that you have professionals explain any report to you, even though it will be in some ways vague. Remember, these were the results of my neuropsychological evaluation. A stroke victim might be given different tests and have different percentiles. So just get the broad picture of the information that the evaluator gives to you.

Work and Homework and Rehabilitation

Transitions of Long Island's team used all these tests and subtest, reports and anecdotal information from Peggy to plan a program for me. There were reports, including a Neuropsychological Evaluation on me, to the insurance company. Transitions of Long Island wanted the insurance company to pay Transitions of Long Island for ongoing treatment for me. Transitions of Long Island's plan was to try to help me to improve my receptive and expressive language skills. They wanted me to improve my processing speed and attention and compensate for my difficulties with recalling information.

In retrospect, it was a substantial task for me but I suspect also for Deena and mostly Peggy. Peggy, Deena, and Debra Benson, Ph.D, wrote four months worth of goals for me, from April to July 2002. I want you to see the path that they planned to take me on so that I could be made "whole". They wrote some short-term goals similar to Individual Education Plans (IEP) in schools for the handicapped. These were my short-term goals:

1. Improve use of compensatory strategies to boost auditory recall of paragraph length material, to 80% over 10 trials

2. Improve attention and concentration

3. Improve speed of processing on written tasks when writing 3-4 paragraph length material

4. Improve reading of words and phrases to 85% over 25 trials

5. Improve ability to identify and self correct errors in written work

6. Improve ability to follow 2 to 3 step verbal directions with 1 repetition at 80% over trials

7. Improve syntactic structures in written work, specifically related to tense

8. Improve word finding to 85% over 30 trials when naming pictures and objects without phonemics cues

9. Improve confrontational naming of objects and/or photos to 80% over 25 trials

10. Improve ability to follow written directions to 90% over 30 trials

11. Improve writing skills to generate words to complete common phrases

12. Improve ability to describe complex pictures in a timely manner with increased specificity

13. Improve organization and follow through with use of memory book on a daily basis by completing 4/5 functional memory assignments a week

14. Incorporate family members in therapy sessions to facilitate education and provide support

Remember, these were my short-term goals and they changed as I improved. Your spouse, significant other or parent will have other short-term goals. You should see them and understand them. Ask the professional who works with your stroke victim what you may and should do to help and what you should not do.

The two samples of exercises among others given to me by Peggy or Deena were to help me fulfill the short-term goal to improve reading words and phrases. They were done at home sometimes and checked at <u>Transitions of Long Island</u>. Look at a sample of a simplistic exercise "Read the Sentences and Indicate the Correct Word" and yet I made three mistakes, I wasn't able to write the correct word for 14 gate, 15 time and 18 people.

Read the sentence and indicate the correct word

1	Eat <u>cake</u>	Cake	Pencil	Ladder
2	Read an <u>article</u>	Pen	Brush	Article
3	Wear <u>glasses</u>	Stone	Glasses	Back
4	Fix your <u>tie</u>	Up	Tie	Owl
5	Push the <u>door</u>	Door	Fork	See
6	Write with a <u>pen</u>	Pork	Pen	Smell
7	Make a <u>wish</u>	Wish	Three	Yellow
8	Sing a <u>song</u>	Song	Tire	Shoe
9	Comb your <u>hair</u>	Hair	Rule	Cup
10	Paint your <u>wall</u>	Horse	Wall	Pig
11	Pay with <u>money</u>	East	Money	Happy
12	Open your <u>teeth</u>	Letter	Teeth	Silver
13	Show a <u>picture</u>	Two	Pepper	Picture
14	Close the <u>river</u> x	Cell	Gate	River
15	Watch the <u>but</u> x	But	Was	Time
16	Cross the <u>line</u>	Cone	Line	Web
17	Weave a <u>rug</u>	Rug	Leg	Car
18	Smile at <u>light</u> x	People	Light	Up
19	Sit in the <u>corner</u>	Corner	Four	West
20	Sweep the dirt	Game	Dirt	Cigar

Look at the simplistic exercise "Read the Phrases and Indicate the Correct Word" and yet I was not able to complete the entire exercise. Sometimes Peggy used a word or two from the exercise/lesson as a method to improve my conversational speech.

Read the phrases and indicate the correct word

1	Cat and <u>dog</u>	Dog	Boy	Friend
2	Warm and <u>cool</u>	Eye	Son	Cool
3	Foot and <u>arm</u>	Good	Arm	Spoon
4	Day and <u>night</u>	Baby	Three	Night
5	Sky and <u>sea</u>	Sea	East	Bread
6	Nose and <u>lips</u>	Lips	Salt	Husband
7	West and <u>east</u>	East	Gas	Right
8	She and he	Meat	He	Girl
9	New and <u>worn</u>	Worn	How	Tea
10	Chair and	Song	Table	There
11	A cup of	Kleenex	Cold	Sugar
12	An inch of	Paper	Spoon	When
13	A bunch of	Carrots	Oil	Glasses
14	A pint of	Cream	Eggs	Carpet
15	A foot of	Wood	Ink	Cheese
16	A spoon of	Bread	Soup	Day
17	A pound of	Turkey	Socks	Chair
18	A dozen	Pepper	Bagels	Three
19	A jug of	Flowers	Work	Water
20	A sink of	Cake	Dishes	Eye

At this point of my rehabilitation I was exhausted. I struggled to fulfill my homework assignments at night. I had to enter data for the schools that I consulted with. After all I had fiscal responsibilities. Peggy was not an ogre but she pushed me as far as possible. Without Peggy this book never would have been written. I know that this book was a product of her professionalism and her tenderness.

She, Peggy, was an enigma. Sometimes she was detached and objective and sometimes delicate and personal but always involved in my rehabilitation. She looked at me in clinical ways every time I went into her office or room. She didn't miss a beat when I spoke with and to her. Did I use more sophisticated words and phrases from one day to another? Did I remember my thoughts after she interrupted me in our conversations? Did I make eye contact as she and I spoke? Did I use tense appropriately at this time of my rehabilitation? I suspected that she asked all the people that I had contact with each day about my speech, conversational speech, and eye contact. I was relieved that she did that. The delicate and personal Peggy knew the names of all my sons, daughter (in-law), my granddaughters, step son and his wife and step daughter and her husband. At the same time Peggy allowed me to vent, probably daily when I think of those 15 months, not at God, but the lack of control of my life and the people I loved.

Physical and Psychological Rehabilitation

It was about this time of the year that I joined the cardiovascular exercise class in St. Francis Hospital and I also entered into psychological therapy. These two activities were made part of my health routine by my doctor and me. My insurer never ever called me or wrote to me to say Don your health policy allows you to join a cardiovascular exercise class and the right to go to psychological therapy and these could be very beneficial for you and you should talk to your doctor about these.

The nurses at the cardiovascular exercise class were very competent. It was a one hour three days a week program for sixteen weeks. My insurer, Empire, paid for most of this service. It was appreciated although I don't know why either Empire or the government didn't pay the whole cost for this physical therapy. How many bombs does it cost to pay for this therapy? How many over run military contacts does it cost to pay for this therapy? How much pork barrel legislation does it cost to pay for this therapy? There was a practice at St. Francis. Nurses took my blood pressure as soon as I entered the gym. That was followed by warm ups. After that I worked out on treadmills, bikes and weights. Next, the nurses took another blood pressure test. More exercise followed and then I warmed down. This was a worthwhile activity for me.

On the other hand the psychological therapy was worthless for me. The therapist was not a Ph.D. I suspect that she was a social worker. The therapist never had a stroke and didn't add anything substantive for me. Perhaps it was because my handicap handicapped me. My thought was that the therapist was not a specialist of strokes. After all, the universities just get their tuition and belt out the degrees. Then clinics, where they work, allow them to be jacks of all trades masters of none. My therapist was a stroke "expert". There was no inclination that the therapist could help me and the couple of things that we talked about were perfunctory.

It took me many minutes and weeks before I knew that this was a waste of time for me and I stopped going. It was just a bad fit but it was important for me to know that this type of help was available should I need it.

Modifying my Medicine

There were mixed thoughts, no, mixed feelings in April 2002 but there was one overriding passion in my makeup and it was to be free, to be free so that no one would have to take care of me, to be free to finally tell myself what I feared and didn't fear including death, and to be free so that I could allow the people closest to me to go on with their lives. On April 1, a Monday, Dale left to go the California to see her daughter. She left for the airport at about 7:30a.m. I went to Transitions of Long Island at about 9:30a.m. Deena was the speech-pathologist who was working with me and four or five patients in the classroom. Suddenly I felt faint, in slow movement I started to fall off my chair. Deena was right there. She called for help. Peggy came and others too. They gave me some orange juice. I told Peggy that Dale was on a plane and not available. Peggy called an ambulance and it took me to North Shore University Hospital. I don't remember much of the first hours in the hospital but that day Dale called me. I don't remember much of our conversation. I don't know how much time past before Peggy reached Anne who reached Dale, but I do remember that Dale wanted me to decide for her whether she should come back immediately to be at my side. There were three instantaneous gut reactions on my part. She needed to make that decision by herself. I was safe in the hospital and Jeff and Anne were around to see me or call me. Also, equally important to me was that my fainting was not a psychosomatic reaction to Dale's trip. That would not be allowed by me for me. The doctors needed to adjust my warfarin medicine I think. I had to stay in North Shore University Hospital for five days before they allowed me to go home. The lesson was not lost on me. I needed to make sure that I took my prescribed medicines daily and if I felt uncomfortable in my body I would call my doctor immediately and if I still felt concerned I would get to his office as soon as possible.

Signs on the Road

Every day when I went to Transitions of Long Island and came home I tried to improve my reading. On Monday, April 8, I drove to Transitions of Long Island following the same route that I took daily only now I was aware that I was trying to read the big red hexagon "Stop" signs on the street corners. At first I stuttered as I looked at the "Stop" signs just as I slowdown to put on my brakes. It must have taken a couple weeks going back and forth to Transitions of Long Island before I was comfortable with seeing the "Stop" signs and saying aloud in my Corolla "Stop". Parallel to this feat were others, but they took more time. It took more time before I was able to sound out the small rectangular red and white "No Stopping Any Time" signs near street curbs. I tripped over my tongue and hesitated on "No" and "Stopping" and "Any" and "Time". It was very difficult for me to remember "Any" and "Time". It took time and patience. Even now three years after my graduation in May 2003 from Transitions of Long Island periodically I have to still stop a moment to read the signs silently. That was true for "East" and "West" signs on or from highways, signs on stores and movie facades.

My Parents Rose and Harry

I don't know the specific date in April nor can I say with certainty that it was in April, I didn't write down the day or date, but it was around April when I stopped at a red light

on Hillside Avenue and Herricks Road going home from
Transitions of Long Island. On the left side of the street
there was a flower store façade with a Rose, the store was
Roses and Stems. I had passed this façade day in and day
out to and from Transitions of Long Island. Somehow I
must have seen the Rose and made some kind of a
connection or two. This time I saw the Rose and I said
Rose, Rose, Rose, Rose and Harry, Harry, Harry, Harry
until the light changed and I said Rose and Harry over and
over until I felt sure that I could say Rose and Harry
fluently. For the first time since my stroke on this day and
time I was able to remember my mother's and father's
names and I cried quietly and soon I howled. I kept calling
my mother's and father's names, Rose and Harry, and then
my Grandfather's and Grandmother's names, Poppa Julius
and Bubby Fanny Fishner, but I always called them just
Poppa and Bubby.

Pictures of my Family

From the first time Dale and I married she made sure that
there were pictures of all five of our children on the walls
and tables and bedrooms. As they grew and married and
had children the number of framed-wood, gold, silver, blue,
glass and other varieties- pictures grew also. I never had
any pictures of my parents or grandparents on the tables or
walls. There were pictures of them in my Bar-Mitzvah
book but before my stroke I looked at the pictures maybe
once or twice every couple of years and then only when I
was alone for a minute or two. This past year, December
2005, I had a printer, Bill, use some techniques and print
copies of my parents and grandparents from my Bar-
Mitzvah book, mounted and framed. They are on the wall
in the living room and I see them every day. One of the
changes that I see in myself is that I need to see daily the
pictures of my blended family from my grandparents,
parents, sons Jeff, Robert, Erick, daughter (-in-law), Anne,
granddaughters Alison, Jessica, Lily, Katherine, nephew
Richard, grandniece Elie, stepson Mark and his wife Dana
and stepdaughter Jill and her husband Julian. My morning

starts and my day ends when I look at pictures on my dresser of Alison and Jessica.

Philosophy

There are limitations, the nature of the stroke, the severity of the disabilities in different domains, for your stroke victim. Within these confines your stroke victim is able to focus on the life that he wants notwithstanding his disabilities. Your stroke victim may have a philosophy, one that says that life goes on, with you or without you. Your stroke victim may strive as hard as possible to make some minimal gains, gains that make people who love her proud of her efforts and appreciative of her selflessness and respect for them so that they may enjoy their daily activities. Or he can die inch by inch and second by second. He can make people who love him miserable, shut off from sunny days, blue skies, and laughter.

Over the past three years, since I graduated from Transitions of Long Island, I visited with classes or took part in alumni events or committees, and I popped in to see Dan and noticed the camaraderie of the people in the cafeteria. Most of these people had a positive attitude, laughing, "talking", "sharing thoughts", helping one another and unless the water at Transitions of Long Island is unique they are able to "talk", laugh, "share thoughts" and help others at home.

At this time I had a full daily schedule, data entry, speech with Peggy, other therapies, business meetings with people and personal worries. All stroke victims have a life with other problems, some more than others, but if they live and they want to be part of life than they have to understand that the ups and downs of life goes on and on, stroke or no stroke, that is the nature of life.

There were Ecclesiastical joys for me from April to July, times for birthdays, Mother's Days, Father's Days, soccer games, and dance recitals. On the other hand some dealt with job, bonuses, insurance, spousal, sibling craziness, in-laws, family illness, psychological and drug problems. That is the real world and that was my real world especially when Erick, in May, went in to <u>North Shore University Hospital</u> for back surgery.

When I was younger, maybe 55 years old, I enjoyed my birthday and Father's Day since they were tied together. Dale barbequed shrimps and or salmon and or London broil with vegetables and sweet corn. She bought a Carvel birthday cake too. Jeff, Anne, Robert, and Erick came over for lunch or earlier dinner.

Strategies for Work

In the spring, somewhere in late April to June, Peggy, because she was the main professional responsible for planning and delivering instruction to me, put together a complex strategy that help me get back to my work as an educational consultant and writer. She saw the big picture, intertwined my necessities, as real as the need for breath, with the foundations, reading, writing and memory skills, needed to help me achieve my objectives.

In the midst of spring Peggy and I talked about my job as a consultant. At that time I was able to pronounce some nouns, verbs and adjectives but I thought they were unintelligible except to Peggy and the people at <u>Transitions of Long Island</u> and my family. I knew that I could communicate some by English language and gestures but I didn't think that I could sustain a conversation in a business meeting. I still stuttered and I couldn't sound out words well. I couldn't repeat a word or phrase that was used in a business conversation. I couldn't follow two conversations at once. I unquestionably couldn't respond to staccato questions. That was my perception at the time but it was not quite accurate.

Peggy and I spoke in class numerous times about my infuriation with my stroke. It had no gender, no distinctive name, no predictability; it was a stroke, just a damn stroke.

I was irritated because it came at a wrong time, can you imagine how absurd, how bizarre, how ludicrous it was for me to think that there was a first-rate time for a stroke. But I did. You see I was so focused and disciplined in my actions and dreams and those dreams were a nanosecond away from reality, one flash burst second dream to reality. In 1986, after several years of experience, I wrote Administrator's Guide To Curriculum Mapping: A Step-By-Step Manual. I showed school administrators and teachers how to use this time-on-task program and the program's benefits. Then I got some contracts. All the work required manual entry, remember, schools didn't give teachers computers at that time. Teachers entered data for time-on-task on a sheet. I inputted these data for an analysis for each and every standard and objective and performance indicator for each teacher. In about 1998 some of the schools had placed computers in each classroom for teacher's use. I put my program in every teacher's computer in the school when possible. Sometimes schools didn't have useable computers for teachers in their rooms but they had computer rooms with my program. By 2000 I knew that I wanted to develop my own website, I could market my program throughout the United States. It was at this time when I had my stroke. This wasn't a first-rate time for a stroke but there is no first-rate time for any stroke.

Bonding with my Son and Nephew

There is a first-rate time for bliss and that is anytime. It was at this time, somewhere in the spring, that my nephew Richard told me that he would develop a website for me and my son Jeff told me that he would help in any way possible and they both talked together and we talked together. It was wonderful. It was gliding on the Rainbow room dance floor with my wife, it was a balmy 80 degree day in Shea stadium in the left field bleachers with my sons eating three pounds of peanuts, 20 pieces of Chicken Delight, 2 hotdogs for each of us, a couple of beers for Jeff and me and a couple of Cokes for Rob and Erick, and some ice cream, it was a walk on the beach in Long Beach Island talking, laughing, stopping, looking, playing and holding hands with Alison and Jessica, it was the sound when Anne calls me Dad. Somewhere in the midst of this stroke of mind I got to feel the ecstasy of my son and nephew, working to help me, to talk with me about my interest, the work of nearly 25 years. We connected man to man, father to son and uncle to nephew. I learned more about their excitements and expectations. We spoke on the phone and we e-mailed one another. Out of the hellish anguish of my stroke came the beauty of my bonding with my son and nephew in ways that I suspect would not have happened but for my stroke. Here was a first-rate time for bliss. Hoist one for my stroke.

Contracts

Peggy was a great cheerleader day in and day out especially when I spoke with her about my need to extend my contract with the Middletown School District and to get a new contract with the Roosevelt School District also. I told her about my trepidations, the stress of the 200 mile drive to and from Middletown, my uneasiness to be in a business meeting, my qualms about my ability to speak so that people could understand me easily and my apprehension about my skills to take notes from a meeting including dates and costs.

Peggy suggested a plan for me. She and I would walk through a mock business meeting; what words would I need to use, what thoughts would I need to get across, should I need to submit a Microsoft Power Point presentation. All of these questions required homework for me. When I say me in reality it meant me and Dale because we spoke daily on all issues. There were my issues, Dale's issues, our issues, and our brood issues. That night I should have marveled about Peggy's teaching skills. You see one of the exercises that Peggy put me through time and time again was the one that required me to give names of animals in a minute or so or words that started with a special letter. For this night I tried to remember significant words for my software program and synonyms such as CMT, time-on-task, horizontal and vertical articulation reports, and input data. Once I remembered one all of the other significant words just flowed out of my mouth. The real hard problem was then to write a series of small paragraphs made up of two or three sentences to express a specific thought. The general idea was that I would read my thoughts. By the time I went to bed that night I knew that I couldn't read the presentation, I just couldn't read precisely and fluently.

The next day we modified the plan. I read the paragraphs. Peggy understood my dilemma at once. She saw other problems too. I was not able to focus on her face when I spoke to her. I couldn't find words when I tried to speak. I stuttered periodically. Peggy and I agreed that if I was more comfortable I should limit my presentations and speak in a conversational style. That was what I did.

I am not sure of all of the dates for meetings with the Assistant Superintendents of Middletown and Roosevelt School Districts. Sometimes I was able to put cursory notations in my day minder calendar but I am not able to understand my cryptic penmanship now. Oftentimes Dale put the information on a wall calendar so that she and I would remember my appointments, medical, professional and personal. In reality, it was another gentle way that Dale helped me to work my way back to health with dignity. She kept another calendar in her colossal teacher union bag but only the mighty could lift it. I found some word files regarding my work with both districts that indicated the original dates and other details and narrowed the dates for these meetings.

As a result of my stroke, planning and strategizing were and are the watch words for any trip, especially a trip of two hours or more. I don't want to hurt myself and I don't want to hurt others so I plan to allow more time to get somewhere at the right speed, about 55-65 miles per hour on highways. Also, I planned for health stops every 45 minutes or there about, to go to the bathroom, get an orange juice and walk a little bit. Dale always packed me a travel care package made up of bottled water, a Ziploc bag full of berries and almond or walnuts, and a piece of fruit. I put in my Kingston Trio, Rod Stewart, Bette Midler, and Fiddler on the Roof CDs and I leave about 9:30 a.m. after morning traffic. I executed my plan when I went to Middletown; Roosevelt was only 15 -20 minutes from my house.

At the end of the day I got both contracts. Although both Assistant Superintendents had different personalities and relationships with me it was clear to me that both of them had to see me as healthy, upbeat, and intellectually sharp able to fulfill any contract better than anyone else. That was what I did. About a week before my meeting with Patricia McLeod at Middletown I got a haircut. I got a good night sleep. I put on my spring multi-colored impressionist tie, Vase de Fleurs by Monet, that Dale got me, and my dark blue stripe suit, a Polo blue shirt that Anne and Jeff got me for either Chanukah, my birthday or father's day, with cordovan wingtip shoes. I felt good and I looked good, yes indeed, I was ready for the meeting. That was not the way I felt prior to the meeting. I suffered. It was Gary Cooper at High Noon except my protagonist was me and my anxiety. Good or bad most of the time prior to my stroke I dealt with painful issues swiftly, oftentimes the choice was not a choice, and can the Pope be anything but the Pope? There was the train; there was the High Noon song, the tempo increases. Will I choke? woo, will I find the words? woo, will I stutter? woo and here comes the train into the station woo, woo, woo. Well, I shot my fear and anxiety. I shot them right in their eyes. Yes I did. My grooming and my clothes did their jobs well. My English and gestures did their jobs well also. A little chat so that Pat could see whether she could understand me and my thoughts. My apparent good health did its job well too. Those were pieces important pieces but the foundation of the building was my software program. The program assisted Maple Hill Elementary School teachers and that improved student test scores by about 14% over two years. That was why I got the contract, quality, accountability and performance

72

but those other pieces were important. The administrators knew me and my program and were ecstatic at tests scores.

Nice Teachers at the Roosevelt School District

Prior to my stroke I consulted with the Roosevelt Union Free School District a district that had severe academic problems. The administration wanted me to help teachers design and develop local curriculum guides that aligned classroom instruction with the New York State assessment examinations and ensure horizontal and vertical articulation of programs. By late spring I met with a recently hired Assistant Superintendent of Curriculum and Instruction. My perception of the meeting differed with reality apparently. That was my thought when I spoke with Peggy the next day. I brought in a prototype of a model of a curriculum guide. The curriculum guides included New York State standards, performance indicators, content, strategies, resources, assessment and timelines, 25 years of experience and insight. The expectations for the faculty were to develop drafts of middle school English, Math, Science, Social Studies and high school English, Math A and Chemistry curriculum guides by the end of the summer. Obviously, my English and my gestures were sufficient to explain my process. I got the contract. Again, the building pieces were there but the prototype curriculum guide, I am sure, helped me to get the contract. It was clear to the administration that the process that I proposed was practical and useable.

In retrospect, there were important lessons from these two meetings for you. Prepare for all meetings. First, meet with people who know your qualifications and competences and had seen the results of your work, which would be true for a multitude of professions and jobs such accountants, doctors, photographers, lawyers, cartoonist, writers, analysts, landscapers, and clowns. After all there was the technological miracle that made the physicists-astronomer, Stephan Hawking, speak and his tenacity to live. I admired the actor, Kurt Douglas, after his stroke when he went on the Larry King television program with his speech limitations. Remember, the Assistant Superintendents and only they, not me, assessed my plusses and minuses for the job and they and only they came to the conclusions that my limited English speech together with gestures would still allow me to do my job splendidly. Please don't sell yourself short, the manager and only the manager can tell you whether there is a good fit.

There was a sixty year old plus man who had a stroke, his speech was severely impaired, he didn't have the benefits of <u>Transitions of Long Island</u> or any other help, and his life was tied to his job as a super Cadillac salesman and within a year or so he died. Some think that he died because he couldn't work as a super Cadillac salesman, he loved those Cadillac's. Would there have been a supervisor who would have seen him has a good fit for his dealership, not as a salesman, but in some way based on his car knowledge, finesse at a salesman and organizational expertise? His family doesn't know because he and they didn't gamble on his expertise and the people in the business who knew him. The worst situation would have been that he got out of his house and spent time with some old friends. They would have talked a little. He would have come out of his stroke closet. The truth be known who knows, so many factors so many dynamics in one person's life.

The Jassie's and a Safe Heaven

The Jassie's were not part of the Catholic, Jewish or Protestant Revolutions or sects, nor fifth columnist, Luddites or Jacobins but were Anne parents and Jeff's in-laws and my granddaughters other grandparents and for this I was grateful. They, Dr. Marvin and Mary Jassie, and their two other daughters, Karen and Susie, and their son-in-laws, David and Mark, made a model family. They were gentle, reasonable, personable, witty and sensible. They lived within no more than one hour away from any of their daughters. Their son-in-laws were marvelous, they had a good sense of humor, they were sport aficionados, all sports all teams. David was a Boston Red Sox, Celtic and Bruins fan and Mark was a Yankee, Nets/Knicks and Rangers/Devils fan. They had their own thoughts on politics and current issues and who they were.

The warmest sensations happened, during June to July, when we got together in Anne and Jeff's house. June was the time for Alison's dance recital. July 4 was Jeff's birthday. There was Mary, with her enticing English accent, and her three daughters, all with her voice, so agreeable, so capable, so strong, so earthy chatting on anything and everything as they prepared appetizers and entrées in the kitchen. Although Anne, Karen and Susie either made cookies, cakes or brought bakery products I salivated for Mary's cakes, strawberry short cake, brownies and jelly rolls. This was one of four or five times that I went off my diet. What put the cherry on the top of this picture was the fact that neither Anne or Mary or Karen or Susie professed proprietary ownership in the kitchen. From the first time we got together at Anne and Jeff's house, maybe eight years ago, they welcomed Dale into the group with all the rights and privileges of the clan and she also chattered and prepared the food and the ubiquitous discussions, chatter and gossip warmed my heart. It was also inviting to hear Jeff, David and Mark shoot the bull about their kids, sports, the stock market and houses, Bush and the Afghanistan war. They were congenial. They liked each other. They cared for each other and their families. Their cheerfulness came through as did their enthusiasm and their passions. The great respect and love for Marvin and Mary from all three son-in-laws was evident. It was a testimony to Marvin and Mary and their daughters who married such sterling men.

They, all of the people, made me comfortable at all times at Anne and Jeff's house. The greeting and good-bye hugs from Mary, Karen and Karen's daughters Jackie and Melanie and Susie and Susie's Daniel had importance to me. Their faces mirrored not some inquisitive expressions, but deep sorrow and empathy. Karen's face had tears etched all-around her eyes and I remembered that vividly and all the Jassie women and men were compassionate. They talked to me, they didn't talk to me, they listened to my questions and answers, they talked to others, they laughed and they did. I was not the center person. I was not the Bar Mitzvah boy in the room. I was not infantized. Their sensitively changed a whale to a fish.

There wasn't any uneasiness for me. David had a great sense of humor and he was a good raconteur. He was lively and compassionate. He would have made a great poster boy for a sports bar advertisement. He was 6'4", athletic, he played basketball at Brandeis and his smile was infectious. Mark was more serious and lower keyed. He was a musician and owned a health store. He sure liked to laugh and was a great audience for Jeff and David. Mark got a lot of pointed one liners. Mark's face was deceptive. Its features were from the 1890s from Paris and Vienna, in the form of Pasteur and Freud. He and I spent about 45 minutes playing ping pong in the basement. Mostly he talked and I laughed at his comments and jokes.

Because it was safe for me I was able to try out my speech and vocabulary. Politics was the easiest issue to talk about and it was always in style. The vocabulary was limited. Bush and Cheney were bastards. That took six words, the tense came naturally. I was not concerned about nuances, oil was oil, liars were liars, and those were two words. Cheney, Rumsfeld and Wolfowitz were murders, three words although it was difficult to say Rumsfeld and Wolfowitz time and again. Falwell, Robertson and Reed, it was difficult to say their names consistently especially when they were championing Israel. Those names just didn't compute with Israel except for their evangelical dogma. My face conveyed all my thoughts so I got more mileage from these eight words. That was enough to keep me in the conversation. It didn't have to deal with tense. I didn't have to use words such as "either" and "comparison". And I didn't have to couple two or more thoughts from literature, articles, and authorities.

The give and take in the kitchen was music in my ears, soft guitars followed by swing. All of the people ate appetizers, drank sangria and walked around the hexagon fixed kitchen island table. They either stood or sat on barstool height chairs. I looked at all of these people in the room and the words by Woody Guthrie's <u>This Land Is Your Land</u> had meaning to me although I couldn't say it or sing it or even remember it. Throughout the appetizer portion of this lunch/dinner Anne and Jeff asked Marvin and me if we had enough to eat and drink. I loved the word "Dad" when they called Marvin and me, same words, same love, same devotion although he was "Poppy" and I was "Grandpa" to Alison and Jessica.

Curriculum Guides for the
Roosevelt Union Free School District

At this period of time, July to August, I had mild-to-moderate apraxia, with halted speech pattern and underdeveloped responses to questions. Yet I was able to show about twelve teachers how to design and organize components of a curriculum guide. In the course of this activity I also grew in ways that I could not in my wildest dreams fantasize. I went outside of my stroke victim box and learned that I cared about other people and issues passionately and that dwarfed myself centered self for hours and hours.

Sorrow takes different forms and regret happens even for stroke victims. I was upset that school administrators had such contempt for the middle and high school academic programs, disrespect for teachers, and disregard for students. In late July until mid August I worked diligently with a nice group of teachers, about twelve in all, but they, for the most part, were regretfully under qualified. They were elementary teachers instead of 7th -12th grade teachers. They were not knowledgeable of content, students, the district's educational resources and the historical perspective for grades 7th-12th. The administration agreed that at least two teachers needed to develop each curriculum guide but that didn't happen in some of the course disciplines. The administration decided that teachers could work at home rather than at school. One teacher rather than a committee would design a curriculum guide. I suggested to the administration that school psychologists should review the content and strategies to ensure that the content and strategies were age appropriate. Teachers and psychologists needed to determine whether the methods used were age appropriate and geared to the ability levels of students. I suggested that the Assistant Superintendent be present at all the curriculum guide workshops. After all, the state education department took over his district and curriculum and instruction made up at least 75% of the district's budget. His presence once a day for a half hour would bring home the importance of this curriculum guide workshop. To my recollection he didn't visit the curriculum guides workshops on any regular basis, never looked at the draft guides daily and never asked questions of all the teachers who wrote the guides.

Notwithstanding these problems these teachers worked relentlessly to develop curriculum guides. Curriculum guides aligned classroom instruction with the New York State assessment examinations. They ensured horizontal and vertical articulation of programs. By the end of the summer we developed drafts of middle school English, Math, Science and Social Studies curriculum guides. We did the same thing for high school English, Math A and Chemistry. These curriculum guides include New York State standards, performance indicators, content, strategies, resources, assessment and timelines.

In spite of all the barriers this group grew academically and intellectually. Although they spent less than three weeks, each day for 5-6 hours, they developed drafts that a representative of the state education department thought was right on target for curriculum guides. To the best of my knowledge, unfortunately, none of the teachers who wrote these guides were ever debriefed by the administration and I was told recently that a new Middle-High School

Principal put in her own programs. She is now gone and the schools are still under the control of the state education department. How sad how regretful for the Roosevelt Free Union School, students and teachers, not just for me. The price of poverty was a stranglehold on schools, teachers and students.

Throughout those three weeks or so I made gains, tremendous gains, gains that were miraculous, gains in self confidence, gains in speech, and gains in focusing my thoughts. I credit this to most of the elementary teachers in this program. These were the very same teachers who were not "qualified" to put together curriculum guides for the middle school, and others with high school experience who worked on high school curriculum guides. But please remember without the help of Peggy Kramer and all the people at Transitions of Long Island and Dale, Jeff, Anne, Alison, Jessica and Pierre Woog I would not have been in this enviable position.

But the linchpin for this was Hannah Hill, a former graduate school pupil of mine, in her 40s, black, with about 20 years of teaching experience. I suspect that her presence gave me instant credibility with the workshop group notwithstanding my handicaps. The group was made up of about 10 women and 2 men. There were Black, Latinos and Whites. They were Catholics, Jews, Muslim, and Protestants. But they were teachers and agreeable people.

I explained to Mrs. Hill and the other teachers the design format and the components of the curriculum guide. There were only 14 words that I needed to use to get my thoughts through to the workgroup, curriculum guides, standards, performance indicators, content, activities, resources, assessments, time, horizontal and vertical articulation and specific. These words were part of my vocabulary for decades and I practiced those words over and over for my presentation.

I showed them a copy of the boilerplate, the design and the components parts of the guide. The boilerplate was pretty clear, however, Hannah, in her subtle and unmistakable manner walked the other teachers though the process when she thought that the others were unclear about the process or details for each of the components. I suspect that as teachers, especially elementary school teachers, their skills were honed and they were able to figure out the correct words and terms that I used. If they didn't there was Hannah, the interpreter.

Nobody knew that I was illiterate at this time. I had some teachers proof the English in all the drafts and I proofed the sequence of the standards. I tried to read all the drafts letter by letter word by word. This exercise was useful and practical for me but it was tedious and emotionally exhausting. I read the drafts every day and night for four hours. When I was drained Dale read the drafts to me also. After I proofed these drafts I explained my concerns to the teachers involved. These were practical applications of goals that Peggy made for me.

There were other benefits for me and those were ancillary to the project but wonderful for my speech. It turned out that there were two people in the group who took exception to the project. One I suspect was upset because she had to proof some of the drafts. The other felt stress, academic and intellectual growth and frustration all at the same time. When I was a kid of 11 or 12 in Brooklyn I went to Hebrew school daily except Fridays and Saturdays after I finished public school at 3 p.m. Every Sunday the Hebrew teacher read us stories about the mythical peaceful village or shtetl of Chelm (not the people in the real town of Chelm that were killed by the Nazis) populated by fools. The first educator would have lived comfortably in Chelm, maybe even one of the elders. The other teacher was on the threshold of her educational evolution. In both cases I was able to practice my conversational speech. Much to my surprise I used words that I had not used since my stroke, but the discussion with the embittered Chelmite was wearisome. How many ways to explain that the school lacked usable practical curriculum guides and students scores on state tests were among the lowest in the state?

I wanted to thank her for the limited conversation with the limited vocabulary yet it improved my vocabulary. The neo-renaissance woman asked why and how. She finally understood the rationale for the process and each of the components. Our exchanges were more substantive. That allowed me to push myself. I learned specific words such an analogy, compare and outcome for our talks. The bottom line was that I enjoyed the daily give and take with these people. They made me feel that they thought I was intelligently and physically competent to battle with me notwithstanding my stuttering and inability to find words to finish thoughts. I loved it.

Conclusion

My neuropsychological report pointed out the constraints of my brain and body but it did not give me a plan or a map so that I could grow in intellectual, arousal and attention, language, memory, visual-spatial and frontal lobe domains at a specific rate. But it did help the professionals at Transitions of Long Island who designed a program for me. There were adjustments, wonderful if not miraculous improvements, because of the expertise of the professionals at Transitions of Long Island, my family, friends and acquaintances and myself. I could see and feel growth. Changes took place in my brain and body in different contexts, times and places. They happened in minuscule ways hardly visible to others and at other times there were obvious gains as I moved through the continuum from stroke victim to stroke survivor.

Checklists

Stroke victim stroke survivor needs to:
1. Push hard to improve their reading, speaking, and writing skills but no more than two hours daily. These are strenuous activities and physically and emotionally draining.
2. Talk daily with their spouse, significant other and other relatives and friends. Tell them to just keep talking for the sake of talking. Never have any one say that they don't talk to their spouse, relative and

friend. The more they talk the more those around them know that they are alive.

3. Ask your doctor about all the kinds of therapies that would help you, as a stroke victim and survivor, such as cardiovascular exercise classes and psychological therapy, to improve your health and then find out if your insurer has to pay for those services. Make sure that any psychologist who calls himself an expert verifies this with documentations and a stroke history personally or in his immediate family.

4. Be sensitive to the changes in your brain and body. Know when you are able to say or feel a new letter, word, and thought. Repeat the new letter, word, and thought over and over until you own them.

5. Look forward to parties with family and friends. You will not be an 800 pound gorilla if you don't want to be one. You can listen to conversations, laugh, smile, be upset and say a word or two or a sentence or two when you and only you want.

Family members need to:

1. Be cheerleaders, encourage your loved one to talk, read, and write and to be part of family events. Go on vacations together. Be a cheerleader but not a drill sergeant. Be supportive but not fearful for your loved one. Be there for him but let him try and if he fails cheer him up. Let him try again and again and again.

2. Understand the limitations that your loved one has at a specific time and place. Those limitations may change but no one can say with certainty when and the degree of change.

3. Be sensitive as much as possible to the changes in your loved ones brain and body. Just know that your loved one's brain and body go through changes and you probably won't know unless he tells you.

4. Know that at this period of time your loved one loves you, appreciates what you have done for him and is thrilled to talk with you and visit places with you, parks, museums, beaches, and movies.

Chapter 4: April-July 2002 - Reading

Preview

This chapter spells out my struggle to relearn to read and the strain to become an outgoing person. In Chapter 3, there was detailed information about my test results, some of which related to my reading abilities by the summer 2002. With hindsight it established a framework so that I could evaluate my progress in reading after five months at Transitions of Long Island. Chapter 4, integrates the application of reading skills learn and practiced at Transitions of Long Island and my tenacity. It specifies the practical minuscule but strenuous accomplishments achieved so that I could become a reader and the secondary benefits derived as I read three books by the end of the summer 2002.

This is a concise chapter but a powerful one and heart wrenching one. It gives you a detailed picture of my struggles to read and my struggle to become an outgoing person. When you read this chapter you will know what you need to do to:

◊ Marshal all your strength when you start your own reading program.
◊ Prepare for the draining, frustrating and taxing daily work that is required for you to become a better reader.
◊ Develop a realistic time frame for you to become a reader.
◊ Understand the mercuric ride that you will go through as you read books meant for kindergarten students to adults. Each of these books that you read will spark off ups and downs for the characters. Some of these books will trigger reminders about your past and in a second see that past. It will vanish in another second but you will have hoped to see that past again.

The Significance of Reading to Me in Perspective

From the time I entered Adelphi College in the halcyon days of 1957 until I had my stroke in February 4, 2002, a time of turbulence, I was a vociferous reader. When I was a freshman it was so exciting for me, for the first time, to know that my thoughts were the same or similar to the opinions of Homer, Socrates and Herodotus. I enjoyed my time with Mark Twain's <u>The Adventures of Huckleberry Finn</u>, Jacques Rousseau's <u>The Social Contract</u>, Thomas Hobbes' <u>Leviathan</u> and John Locke's <u>Two Treatises of Government</u>. It was electrifying to read about the evolution of nation states, the cynical motivation of the John Hancock Insurance Company in Britain in the 1840s to insure children who worked in the mines, a couple of pence to insure their burial and the push and tug that molded The United States of America, the highest ideals and the most despicable corruption of the political soul. I was hooked on reading although I had just put my toe in the academic waters. Reading stimulated me; it seeped into every cell, niche and granny

After I earned my BA degree I read daily every day week days and weekends for about four to ten hours. You see I worked as either an elementary, middle or high school English or social studies public school teacher. Once I had a second full time job after school as a recreation leader. That job ended at about 11p.m. When I no longer worked as a full time recreation leader I worked as a recreation teacher sometimes from about 6 pm to 9 pm in schools. After 1965 or so I worked at an adjunct history instructor or assistant professor at City College of New York (CCNY) and Queens College. I continued my education at the same time as I earned my MA in European and American History from CCNY and my doctoral degree (Ph.D) as a full time student from The City University of New York with a major in Latin American History and minors in European and American History.

There were books and articles to read, there were books when I awoke there were books when I went to bed and there were articles in the bathroom. Every Saturday and Sunday I went to the New York Public Library at 42nd Street and Fifth Avenue to read books and articles from the stacks, this was pre-computers in the library. In my mind, after 6 pm on weekends, there were only graduate students and degenerates in the library and as I spent more time in the library it became more difficult for me to distinguish one from another. Seven days a week I read and read. During this time, for graduate school courses alone, I imagine that I read about 500 books fully and about 2500 books partially and thousands of pages of reports and journals. Once my doctoral dissertation subject, <u>Juan B. Justo: An Argentine Socialist</u> was approved I suspect that I read about 35000 pages from English and Argentine Spanish books, newspapers, and journals. The time spent in researching, analyzing and writing my dissertation was one of the most wonderful exercises for me. As wonderful as this experience was I never went back into the 42nd street library again except once or twice and that was for less than ten minutes or so to show someone the building, my sons, Dale, and friends from out of state.

This kind of reading intensity, depth and breathe was unique to my graduate days. After those days I worked as a public school administrator, college/university assistant/associate education professor and educational consultant. I read daily but the subject matter was less intellectual. The educational books and articles, especially for administrators, were often dreary, part of a fad such as whole language and the new math, written by disciples who brought nothing new to the table. During this period I read the current literature in educational administration and especially in curriculum. The truth be told there were a couple of attention-grabbing books and articles but not many and the rest were copycats with a change here and change there. I say that knowing that I authored a couple of education administrator books and wrote about ten articles most of which dealt with special education. I did read paperback books such as Clancy, Gresham, and Crichton, for relaxation and sleep.

Transitions of Long Island and Reading

I was a reader and reading was integral to my life before my stroke, it was colors to an artist and notes to a composer, and water to a swimmer. I needed to become a reader again after my stroke. At the outset when I came to Transitions of Long Island I "told" Peggy that I needed to relearn reading and she understood this and worked to make it happen. It was difficult to make me a reader again. There were the classes with Peggy and the exercises daily. I got good support from Dale. Jeff and Anne were always encouraging. Those who loved me would disagree before and after my stroke that I had a good brain. They do agree now that my recuperation was luck and hard work.

In hindsight I credited my reading growth to the disciple learned in my doctoral program and my work ethic; hard work, daily work, pushing myself, pushing to go to another level, in other words to work like an overachieving ant. I couldn't conceive that I had to have a plan, a methodical plan. I couldn't even think about articulating a plan to myself. I couldn't formulate a one sentence outline that I could read. And yet that was what I did, not systematically but piecemeal, piece by piece.

In retrospect there was a daily schedule. I allowed myself to read daily, to read aloud to myself separately from anyone for about two hours, sometimes as much as four hours. There was a break, a 20 to 40 minute walk, so the letters and words that I just learned and read would become part of my brain and my speech. Then I took a nap, a nap for about one hour around noon, so I was big on naps, I loved my naps. When I awoke, some of the words that I had struggled to pronounced while I read, now, I could say them fluently, not all of them but some of them. That was my daily plan.

I started to read as a child learns to read from the beginning, the two or three word sentences, the ones that they can remember by heart, the repetition from one line to another line, the ones that have the same sounds, roots, hit, bit, fit and kit. That was my reading material around March to April or May.

My First Book-Wayside School

My first real book was a 4th grade level reader, the <u>Wayside School</u>. I bought it at Barnes and Nobles adjacent to <u>Transitions of Long Island</u>. A saleswoman helped me to pick out the book. She walked me around one of the aisles where there were many elementary age books and she told me about some of the authors and her opinions of them. I told her, in a low soft voice and with minimum words with a hint of a stammer that my granddaughter, Alison, was about four years old and I wanted to read the book to her and to have her read the book by herself and to me in time. It was a plus that the title was the name of Alison's school-that was a big plus for Alison and one of the characters in the book was "Alison". I was eager to start reading the book as soon as I got home. I wanted to be sure that I would be able to read the book before Alison could and I couldn't. So I started to read at once and it was challenging.

I knew the alphabet letters although I didn't feel comfortable about saying them aloud or in my mind because I couldn't say the letters in order if I started reciting the alphabet after the letter C. I didn't have a handle on the sounds and I couldn't sound out words easily. Peggy gave me a copy of a <u>Newsday</u> article, from June 6, 2000, which correlated a letter to an item such as A to an automobile with a picture of an automobile and told me to try hard to memorize the article.

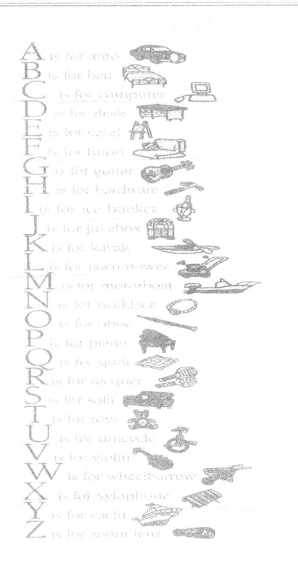

A is for auto
B is for bed
C is for computer
D is for desk
E is for easel
F is for futon
G is for guitar
H is for hardware
I is for ice bucket
J is for jukebox
K is for kayak
L is for lawnmower
M is for motorboat
N is for necklace
O is for oboe
P is for piano
Q is for quilt
R is for racquet
S is for sofa
T is for toys
U is for unicycle
V is for violin
W is for wheelbarrow
X is for xylophone
Y is for yacht
Z is for zoom lens

The first couple of pages of the <u>Wayside School</u> were tough for me. There were new names, names that I couldn't pronounce or sound out effortlessly, names of the teachers and students. There were words that I worked hard to sound out, letter by letter, with different pronunciations. I tried different inflections on a word until I was able to pronounce the word correctly.

It was difficult and required everlasting time, it took about an hour to read the first page, but it was worthwhile and necessary for me to improve my reading. It took me about two or three weeks to read this book. As I read the book I was able to pronounce more of the student names by sight, many words were repeated from page to page and from chapter to chapter and as new words came in play I was able to make usage of clue words. I even laughed about the humor of the book, which was an unexpected pleasure. Please remember that I had to start at the beginning of any sentence if I had any problem with a word in the sentence. It was not unusual for me to go back to a sentence four or five times before I was able to start a new sentence. It was also true that sometimes I had to go back a number of times to the beginning of a sentence because I forgot the gist of the sentence. Sometimes I couldn't repeat the pronunciation of a word even though I just read the word on the previous sentence. But I completed the book and I was proud.

The Navajo Reservation-<u>The Wailing Wind</u>

Soon as I finished <u>Wayside School</u> I bought a new book, a book by an author that I read over the years, Tony Hillerman. The book was <u>The Wailing Wind</u>. I liked Hillerman because he wrote about the Navajo Reservation. I lived for two years in Kayanta near Monument Valley, a place that he noted in his books. His books were readable, the kind of books that I read to go to sleep or at the beach. I liked his characters, Lieutenant Joe Leaphorn and Sergeant Jim Chee of the Navajo Tribal Police. He provided a panoramic view from Window Rock to Ship Rock to Monument Valley to Tuba City. His books gave me some insight to Navajo beliefs and shaman-medicine men.

I felt the growth of my reading in my brain. I couldn't explain the progress but it was there, it was words in my mind, it was thoughts that I had. I felt it in my brain so clearly and yet it was so elusive. I knew that I moved to another level in reading in my brain. There were words such as "as", "at", "for" and "from" that were read as "as", "at", "for" and "from". They were not read one letter by one letter and then sounded out. No, I could say those words in one felt swoop. That was a tremendous accomplishment for me in late spring early summer.

For some reason or other I couldn't pronounce the acronym of FBI, I just couldn't say FBI fluently. I had to go to the beginning of the sentence again and again and say "F", then "B", and "I" and then say the acronym FBI. Perhaps it was because the FBI agent in the book, Osborne, personified the racist attitudes of the white male FBI. By the way that was true of the acronym CIA when I read a line from the New York Times. Maybe that was an emotional reaction to the times in which we live in. I was able to pronounce Joe Leaphorn and Jim Chee easily after one or two times but not the titles of Lieutenant and Sergeant. I got tongue twisted but by the end of the book those titles rolled of my tongue smoothly.

On the other hand I still had to plug away like a broken swaybacked old mare to sound out a word, letter by letter, until I was able to pronounce the word. There were unsaid words also of my physical and emotional stress. Yet when I finally could say the word I felt like a young man with great energy, excitement and hope, it was the spring of my youth again. But the next unknown word brought me back to the emotional roller coaster. Remember, these words were not difficult words or unique words. It would have been easy for an eighth grader to spell and pronounce the words. I couldn't do that at that time. It was letter by letter until I could pronounce the word. It was still difficult for me to sound out the letters in a word and my mind and my eyes focused only on one letter or word at a time but never ever on more than one word at a time, the rest of the sentence didn't exist. Imagine how difficult it was for me to deal with any polysyllabic words. It took a yeomen effort for me to pronounce the last syllable.

One of the secondary or tertiary benefits of reading Hillerman's The Wailing Wind was my remembering life at Kayenta and the vast ocean like desert on the Colorado plateau and the tranquility of Monument Valley. Other names and places burst out from my brain and once in awhile from my mouth also, well not a gust more like trickle, but when there was no movement before it felt like an eruption. There was Ron, Blabe, Bill, Cindy, Paula, Gary, Ken, Yassie, and Lin and people with Navajo names such as Begay, Charlie, Bitsuie, Tsosie and Etsitty. There were kids such as Ronald Young and Susie Yellowhair. I tried to spell their names in my mind and I couldn't spell their names aloud, maybe I was able to spell one name maybe. I wasn't able to describe them orally but in my mind, in a fleeting second, there they were and then they vanished from my mind. There were the coaches, what were their names, the guy who played for Iona High School in New Rochelle, New York, Ed Robinson, and his cute wife and their newborn baby boy. Why can't I remember the name of the teacher who was a former Marine officer (that was what I was told), who had a role in explaining the tragedy at the Ma Lai Massacre (that was what I was told) to the newsmen at the time, a low keyed quiet polite person who kept to himself and his wife and their adopted Navajo son (that was what I was told), one who could destroy any man with his hands, but a gentle man a good man? I liked him and respected him I just didn't know him well.

I just didn't remember his name at the time and that was true for the rest of the faculty. There were the two Navajos, Gilbert and Julius, interpreters who explained life on the reservation to me, the fine distinctions, the culture and politics, day in and day out so that I could become an effective high school principal. There were the old Navajo men proud in their military uniforms, most of them served in the marines or army, when I had them in for an auditorium gym program on either December 7th or for Memorial Day. They were superb, heroes all, Americans.

There was the sight of Mormons proselytizing at a school meeting, a Board of Education meeting, their zeal was unwavering. They wanted to convert the Navajos to the Church of Jesus Christ of Latter-day Saints. They tried to convert me.

There was the majesty of the Grand Canyon, Goosenecks Canyon, and the slow moving San Juan River near Mexican Hat. But there was Kennocott Mine on Black Mesa and the oil, gas, and mineral conglomerates that wanted to get a piece of the wealth under the land. There was the hustle and bustle of the supermarket in Flagstaff a 150 miles away from Kayenta. There was the quintessential symbol of corporative America, the Holiday Inn, at Kayenta and the timelessness of the East and West Mittens in Monument Valley. There was the family style meals and solitude of Goulding and the Dairy Queen in Tuba City near the Hopi reservation. There was the capital of the Navajo reservation at Window Rock and the historic Anasazi ruins at the Canyon de Chelly near Chinle. Then there were the words that said reservation to me; yaateeh, The Dine, chapter house, sand painting, donkeys and horses, pinon nuts Black mesa, fried bread, BIA, sandstorms, hogens, Copper Canyon, turquoise and silver jewelry, woven blankets, sheep, mutton slew and sandstones. But there were doctors, teachers, miners and small businessmen in Kayenta. They were symbols of the non Navajo world with its positive and negative features. I suspect I have never been in an area that had so many people with graduate degrees per population.

Reading Hillerman brought out all these memories, memories that would have been dormant if not lost, reminiscences that opened more of the doors of my mind. My mind remembered. There were fleeting recollections and if they vanished I knew that they would come back to me, when I wouldn't know. I knew that I moved up to another level in my brain. That was what reading did for me and that would have been sufficient for me at that time. But that was a long long way from my ability to synthesize the solitude and beauty of Monument Valley, the Long Walk, Kit Carson and the Massacres of 1863 and a good man who came home from the Ma Lai Massacre to live in Kayenta. It was not possible for me to analyze the teachers in the Kayenta. They came from New York, Chicago, Philadelphia, Indianapolis and Los Angles. They came from small cities and villages. They came to help Navajo kids learn skills and competences needed to deal with the larger society outside the reservation. But it was a good start and I was excited and that was what reading did for me.

Gentle People-<u>Walk to Remember</u>

Somewhere in the late spring or early summer my wife, Dale, suggested to me that I might want to read a Nicholas Sparks book and off we went on Saturday morning to Barnes and Nobles to look for a book for me, a book by Sparks, a large book with big print. It would be a Dale book, a "chick" book, and it was. The book was <u>Walk to Remember.</u> It was a sensitive picture of the metamorphosis of a young seventeen year old boy/man, Landon Carter of Beaufort, North Carolina. Dale and I had been in Beaufort, North Carolina before my stroke. I got a speeding ticket there and I had to send in my check to Judge George Washington something (that was close).

This book was the right book for me at the time. It had new words, words that I had not used since my stroke, idioms, polysyllabic words, words that denoted comparisons. It had compassion, friendship, youthful and mature love, emotion, laughter, pain, piousness and leukemia. I still had to sound out words, letter by letter, until I was able to pronounce the word. I was able to say more words effortlessly, my vocabulary increased, each book increased my vocabulary. Yet I still didn't feel comfortable with the alphabet. Sometimes I couldn't remember the order of the letters and I had major trouble with the sounds of letters. But there was a linear progression, the more books I read the more words I would know and the more words I knew the more I would learn with much less difficulty. Once I was able to say the words and idioms effortlessly in my mind and repeated them orally over and over by myself my speech improved also but that took time.

Remember, there was minuscule growth daily at least that was how it felt in my brain. The reader needs to know the essence of the word "repetition". Repetition means that I still have to sound out some words after four years. Repetition means that periodically, I still have to reread a sentence over and over after four years. Repetition means that I still don't know words by sight after four years. Repetition means that I still don't read well silently. I am not able to pronounce polysyllabic words in my brain silently. After four years, my sight and brain run at different speeds. Now you can understand the reason that I tell you my reading and memory skills from book to book and the secondary and tertiary benefits that I gathered from each book.

The Sparks book exposed emotion, the tender soft feelings of teenage love. There were the raw cuts that rip your insides out when a "healthy" twenty to forty year old loved one dies. This book had a special vocabulary, a different vocabulary, than the other books. It used words and ideals of family, picket fences, school activities and churches. There were tears of love for a child, a child's desire to shelter a father, a journey to manhood, limited time on earth and the need to put in perspective ones fears for material welfare. There were the push and pull of unattached freedom and responsibility. There were feelings for a love one with a deadly illness that has limited times on earth and needs assistance to get around. These words and thoughts unleashed memories and these memories helped me to become more "whole".

The Sparks book allowed me to vent ostensibly against the characters but in reality I cried not for characters in a book but for me daily, quietly, privately and passionately on the couch, in bed or in the bathroom. There were mercurial laugher and wailing. I laughed and cried simultaneously. I didn't know why but I did in a tweak of an eye. I laughed with Landon Carter when he laughed at the piousness of Jamie Sullivan, the minister's daughter. I would never laugh at that sentiment and yet I did. I remembered my first love and her idiosyncratic beliefs and thoughts and my awkwardness. I felt sorry because I never saw the girl as she matured into a woman sure of herself.

Landon and Jamie become friends, sweethearts, lovers and spouses by the end of their senior year in high school. I laughed and cried when they became friends, sweethearts and lovers but I bawled when Landon learned that Jamie had leukemia. I thought that Dale and I had the most wonderful courtship with music, dancing two to four times a week. We held on to each other for our life. There were flowers and passionate love every day. There was laughter and friendship. That courtship lasted fifteen years until my stroke.

I have known the death of loved ones. I knew it from the vantage point of a teenager and a young man and now. My mother died from lipoids, she died at forty-five years old. There was the time when I prayed every second. I hoped for miracles but there wasn't any miracle. She died a painful death. Each day I changed a little bit. I worried about my mother. Then I worried about my mother but I needed to get some sleep and food. I worried about my mother but I needed to get some sleep and food and I had to deal with work. Then I worried about my mother but I needed to get some sleep and food and I had to deal with work and I wanted to spend time with my wife and son. Ultimately there was a metamorphosis from worrying about my mother to a justification for my mother's death for a multitude of reasons, end the pain, my mother's wishes, waste of money and my own mortality and life was passing me by.

The truth is that there isn't a right or wrong answer and I hate that kind of ambiguous answer, those are the words of our psycho social worker world, but it's true in a world populated by free matured spouses. There are many spouses who have hung in with their spouses especially in the twilight of the first year after the stroke. I have always loved Dale not just because she is my wife and I am her husband but I understood that it was a heart wrenching decision she and only she could make. I know that she knows that I know that. She also knew that I would not want her to stay with me out of pity, probably because I didn't see myself as pathetic in any way or shape. There is more than that to me and that was true right after I came home. Because she made her decision, for which I am grateful in so many ways, we have four beautiful granddaughters and a grandson and I love her more than I did before and I loved her so much. I want to live. Now I see myself in my mirror; my hair is whiter than pepper. I am twenty five pounds heavier than I was at college with more fat. I no longer play basketball or run competitively or swim with power. The juices that flew freely prior to my stroke now are treasured and appreciated.

And yet I don't feel that I am old, not at all. I have all kinds of dreams and plans. I treasure my time with Jeff, Anne, Alison and Jessica. I want to see Rob and Erick happy. I want to see what will become of all my grandchildren. I adore the times that Dale and I dance and I feel her arms on the nape of my neck, the feel of her body, her movements and the to and fro of her hips. Dale allows me to make her laugh and she allows me to be there when her adult kids screw up. I love her dinners. She gives me a look over when I go to a business meeting. Dale makes sure that the tags on my suites, jackets, pants, and shirts are off. Her soft hand caresses my neck and puts tee shirt tag back in the shirt.

There were many people that I saw at Transitions of Long Island who too had spouses and families who made efforts, successful efforts, to reorganize their daily lives. Periodically, I have seen Dan. His wife and his daughter-in-law took him to Transitions of Long Island and back to his home. He and his wife periodically go on vacations. I saw a woman with three children who was in the inpatient hospital for about a half a year. Her husband was there for her and I saw him with her at an alumni meeting. Look I don't know the relationships in each of these cases but there were attempts to try to get on with their lives.

The Internet and the New York Times

I used the internet to improve my reading skills especially when I read the editorial articles daily in the New York Times. Peggy encouraged me to read articles, not necessarily in the Times, and write an article about what I read. Initially, I wrote four or five word sentences with no sense of tense. She brought me a book, The Dictionary of Cultural Literacy, for my birthday on June 17th, and with one felt swoop she made me cry with tears of laughter and genuine hope. It had encapsulated, in 575 pages, the highlights of world and United States of America history, literature, politics, social sciences and nature sciences. Although I don't know when my thought process started but it had something to do with the book Peggy gave me. This book that Peggy gave to me showed me the difference between a full healthy human being and human beings whose social senses were impaired some moderately some severely; by that I mean that reading, writing, and speaking are social communicative skills also.

Movement From a Stroke Victim to a Stroke Survivor

People who have strokes are socially withdrawn people. I moved away from the world of silent people to talkative people. I was not a victim day in and day out. I hated being pigeonholed as a victim. I lacked communicative skills. I hated that truth but I was not a victim twenty-four hours a day. I tried to help myself when possible. The more I was able to read or hear about events I was able to be part of the outgoing world. The book that Peggy gave me triggered names of events and people. That allowed me to remember some analogies with historical events and people, not many but one or two. They vanished too quickly from my mind but sometimes I made use of them.

In 2000 C-SPAN's Washington Journal had Mrs. Cheney on to take calls from viewers. I was one of the callers. I told her that I was sure that the Bush team would go to war against Iraq. Oil would be the motivating key for the war and her husband's former company Halliburton would make a bundle off the war. I tell you that because I am not clairvoyant or a Monday morning quarterback. It was surprising to me that so few in Congress and the media failed to understand the Bush-Cheney mentality. I was and am a political junky and I was and am convinced that the whole Bush team should be put in jail for the murder of all American and Iraqi old and young men, old and young women, and children who died in Iraq. I tell you this, not because I want you to share my beliefs, but to understand my choice of articles and writers.

My favorite writers were Maureen Dowd and Frank Rich. Maureen Dowd and Frank Rich dealt with the painful consequences of the Bush regime at the time. John Ashcroft eroded constitutional rights. There was the fiasco of Mr. Mueller's FBI and Mr. Tenet's CIA. There was Vice President Cheney's un-American remark that people who challenge the Bush administration's Mideastern policies were unpatriotic. There were Bush's evangelical crusades for Christendom against Osama bin Laden's fanatical Muslims. Their criticisms were astute, detailed, painted with humor, wit, and absurdity. Their vocabulary pinpointed the essence of Bush and his team. On one hand there were the dangers of unbridled ambition and contempt for truth. On the other hand the Bush-Cheney team had limited understanding of history and unlimited corporative money. What a dangerous combination for the United States of America and the rest of the world.

These articles gave me words that were useable and practical for me such as Cairo, President, Mubarck, that, escalations, Egyptian, intelligence, officials, Osama bin Laden, denied, plots, Judiciary, freewheeling, finger pointing, cliché, carnage, fanatical, Islamic, zealots, and annihilated. It took time for me to pronounce each of these words but the limited scope of the topic, Bush, allowed me, once in a while, to make some guesses of words once I knew one word in a sentence. Once I knew the important words, pronouns, verbs, and adjectives, they were repeated over and over again in the article. The articles that I read gave me instant gratification. By instant gratification I mean that I was able to finish an article in about an hour or an hour and half.

These articles permitted me to become part of the "talkative" world, a word here and a word there and I was part of the club. I mingled. I put in my two cents about the war against Islamic fanatics, the tense might have been wrong but the substantive thoughts were clear. There were broken sentences, not even sentences, but phrases, stuttered phrases. Yet, at those moments I was transformed from a marble statute fixture, noticed in the abstract but not thought about from eyes that drifted away rather than looking at me directly, to a thinking human being with blood and feelings. I had to be measured and evaluated for my thoughts and humor and even sometimes answered and questioned. That was what The New York Times and Maureen Dowd and Frank Rich gave me.

Television

After my stroke I paid more attention to my television than before my stroke and that helped me to become a better reader and a better "talkative" person. That encouraged me to go into the outgoing world. At the outset I just wanted to understand the sounds that came from the television. I made sense of some words and sentences but not all of them. The sitcoms were the easiest to understand, a combination of simplistic themes and slapstick comedy. A couple of the new sitcoms were appealing as were some reruns of classics like MASH and Gunsmoke. By spring or early summer I focused on news programs especially CNN world news. I wanted to know the latest news initially to parrot the words and thoughts that I thought I heard back to Dale every evening and the following morning to Pierre and then to Peggy. These were the three people who spoke with me daily about my obsession with politics. By the time I spoke to Peggy I knew whether I added new words and idioms to my vocabulary and whether I moved up to another level of intellectual sophistication; could I use the words fluently and appropriately. Every day I watched and listened to CNN alone. I said aloud words over and over that the news commentator used. Sometimes I repeated a word at least five times before I stopped. I did that until I just couldn't do it any more for the day. Sometimes I tried to spell some of these words but from my recollection I didn't do well, the problem was that I had memory problems.

The more I watched CNN the more I was aware of the scroll on the bottom of the television picture. The scroll included the highlights of the news, sports results, and weather. The weather included the temperatures of different cities and showed them in degree numbers. Initially, I was able to read one or two words by the time the scroll past from left to right on my screen. It took a great deal of focus to read the one or two words on the scroll on the screen. Once I focused on the scroll I wasn't able to watch or hear the commentators or the clips of the hell in Afghanistan and later in Iraq. It was demanding for me to read aloud the degree numbers from the scroll on the screen. It was difficult for me to go from the 20's to the 50's and the 30's to the 60's and say the numbers aloud.

Although CNN was my television choice for the news I did surf from channel to channel when I got up in the morning. I jumped from CBS to NBC to FOX to ABC. It gave me a fix about the important news for the day and the day's weather prediction. That took me about three or four minutes. I surfed to MS-NBC and the Imus program, C-SPAN and C-SPAN 2. Those programs gave me a better understanding of the political issues that were relevant for that day. The Imus program had politicos whose thoughts I wanted to hear and the intermittent unusual questions from Imus that elicited an answer that revealed some nuance that I didn't know. As a result of my surfing it became clear to me, although my observations were not clinically sound, that the time scroll for different television channels had different speeds. CNN and MS-NBC slowed down the scrolling so that a handicapped person would have a better chance to read the information on the scroll. It was maybe a second difference compared to the other channels but it made a difference.

Conclusion

Initially, my reading goals may not have been lofty to others but they were to me. I had a passionate hunger to read to my granddaughters, Alison and Jessica. I did not want to be illiterate and at best pitied and at worst shamed, I did not want to be humiliated in my own mind by the fact that I couldn't read for the first five months after my stroke. I just did not want to be embarrassed because I could not read. In retrospect, I was motivated to push myself farther than I could have imagined and endured the distressing, exasperating, draining, lonely times needed to become a reader.

As I inched along I had my own daily proof that I was on the road to recovery. The first word that I could read took me from a perpetual stroke victim to a "talkative" person with thoughts and character, a human being that others had to "hear" and "listen" to. With each word, sentence, paragraph, page, article and book I was transformed into another person one that could share cursory thoughts and ideas. Reading triggered my brain to remember emotions, events, issues and people. Once I was able to communicate with words, thoughts and ideas, as shallow as they were, I was part of the outgoing world with my own personal freedom. The importance of reading was life itself.

Checklists

You, as a survivor, need to:

1. Be aware of the appropriate grade level to start your reading program and the understanding that you move up by little increments.

2. Make sure that you know the details about the difficult work that you and only you must do to become a reader again
   ◊ go through the word letter by letter until you are able to pronounce the word,
   ◊ pronounced fluently all words aloud
   ◊ give yourself time to pronounce idioms and polysyllabic words
3. Plan to read daily for two hours
4. Understand that words beget new words, sentences beget new sentences and paragraphs beget new paragraphs. That is how you will become a reader.
5. Ponder paragraphs that you read and ultimately you will produce your own essays or articles from your own thoughts.
6. Acknowledge that there were times, especially when you read, that was one of the wonderful magical moments, to ponder the memories of the past with hazy recollections of people and events.

Spouse and Friend need to:

1. Encourage your spouse/friend to read. Please don't harp on him. Let him know that you are supportive. Leave some newspapers and magazines around for him to skim.
2. Indicate to your spouse/friend that you want to understand the work he has to go through to read one word.
3. Let your spouse/friend share his thoughts with you on the words learned and the sentence or paragraphs read.
4. Don't continuously correct his usage of tense or pronunciations. He will let you know when he is comfortable with your corrections. Make sure that you are not using corrections as a means of humiliating and or patronizing him. Remember, he is an adult with an adult vocabulary stuck in his brain and he is trying hard to become an outgoing person.

Chapter 5: August-October 2002 – I Could

Review

This chapter uses the results of my psychometric tests as a base to observe my actions over three months and the decisions made by <u>Empire</u> and <u>Transitions of Long Island</u> to reduce my time in therapy. It covers my vacation with my family at Long Beach Island, New Jersey and my consultancies in Middletown, New York. It details the tedious, demanding work to read, relearn writing and singing songs.

Within each of these actions there were wonderful events that gave me hope and comfort. It was the cheek to cheek contact daily with my granddaughters in Long Beach Island and the love they gave me every time they called me "Grandpa". It was the fact that the rest of the people of Long Beach Island saw whatever they wanted to see in me, most of the time, if not all of the time, it was a nice guy. It was the pride I felt when I completed a day's work at the Middletown School District. There was my knowledge that I achieved a higher and greater reading sophistication than I thought was possible after I had my stroke. There was the thrill I felt when I sang songs with other stroke and brain trauma survivors. And one of the most incredible achievements of this period, only about four months after my stroke, when I couldn't write a word, I was able to write a very very simple sentence, a two word sentence, an amazing miracle, that gave me more control and power over my life.

This chapter was part of my ongoing struggle to improve my life. It was for the most part positive although there were one or two black marks that dotted the skies. When you read this chapter you will be better prepared to:

◊ Deal with your insurance company before they wean you off from your therapist.

◊ Decide the multitude of joyful tasks that are up to you, babysitting your grandchildren, vacations, exercising, reading, listening to music, seeing movies at the theatre, working, and writing. Make a realistic schedule, the amount of time that you can spend with your grandchildren before you are exhausted or the amount of time that you can sit and write in one shot.

◊ Delineate the tasks, time and energy needed to write. Once you write you will know that writing is control and power.

Testing and Empire Insurance Company August 2002

August 2002 was when my insurance provider, <u>Empire</u>, and <u>Transitions of Long Island</u> decided that it was time to wean me from <u>Transitions of Long Island</u> and Peggy and the other people that I saw daily. They weaned me slowly. I saw Peggy three times a week for one hour daily until January 2003.

Peggy tested me on August 8, 2002. She indicated that I complained about my slowed speech, difficulty with comprehension and slowed processing. She noted that I demonstrated a mild-to-moderate apraxia. Her findings about my Expressive Language Skills included poor eye contact during conversation, halted speaking pattern, word repetition on initiation (e.g. it a, it a, it a) during a description, verbal repetition of target sentences and latency of responses. Her Receptive Language Findings for me indicated that my writing was legible with defects, with important content words absent, with sub clausal syntactic structures and relevant yet incomplete content. She noted that I had difficulty with written narrative skills and comprehension of complex ideation. Peggy recommended that I get speech therapy five times a week for one hour a day. Her short term goals for me were to improve eye contact during spontaneous conversation, verbal fluency, verbal specificity, speed of processing on complex tasks, writing skills (e.g. semantic and syntactic structures), written language from clauses to simple and complex sentence structures and follow through with recommended strategies.

That August day teemed with uncertainty and hopeful anticipation. It was unsettlingly to say the least. Was I a snake's slough discarded or a healthier bear that grew during hibernation? It took me a day or two to decide that I grew but how much and how much more would I be able to grow if I didn't work with Peggy daily. At that thought I fumed at Empire. What gave Empire that right to decide that I should be only half a man when with more speech therapy maybe I could be made "whole"? Who were these people, these unknown people, these faceless people who screw with my life, who I never met, or talked with?

My frustration with Empire gave way to my belief in myself not right way but slowly as the days passed from August 2002 to May 2003. I saw growth in my mind's eyes. It was the new words that I used. There were the extended conversations with family members, friends and acquaintances. There were books that I read. I got consultant contracts. I traveled by car and train to client sights. I slept the Holiday Inn at Middletown for two days twice monthly for six or seven months. There were reports that I wrote and advice that I gave to administrative personnel. I went on vacations with loved ones and traveled to Florida and California.

August 2002-Vacation at Long Beach Island

August started with a brilliant exhilarating bang. We, Dale, Jeff, Anne, Alison, and Jessica, I line them up as chicks whenever I write about them together, went to Long Beach Island, New Jersey, for our annual summer vacation. It had been an annual vacation for three years. It was one of the highlights of my year if not the highlight, and this vacation meant so much to me. Now this is not just an annual vacation but tradition. This year (2006) when the adults questioned the benefits of the Long Beach Island trip my granddaughter, Alison, eight years old, piped up with her objections to that suggestion, she spoke for Jessica also. She said that it was a tradition, she looked forward to the vacation, and she liked to spend time with Gram and Grandpa. And if that's not loving, then God didn't make little green apples.

How beautiful life was in August. I looked around and saw Dale in bed with me. That was a moment of serenity and beauty. The sun broke through the primordial darkness and dawn held a new day for me. I breathed the aroma of the salt ocean from the porch. There was Alison. She was up at 7 a.m. There was her musty morning glow as she saw me on the porch and she came over to me so that I could kiss her on the top of her head. We talked. It was a free flow conversation. We played checkers as we talked. I gave her a buttered bagel or cereal; I didn't do that every day, maybe once or twice. Sometimes she and I took a two block walk over to the deli and bought bagels, coffee and the newspaper for Dale, Anne and Jeff; sometimes, once or twice. The chatter, once everyone was up, was euphony of love. Anne and Jeff wanted Alison and Jessica to know Dale and me as people who loved them. I wanted them to know that I loved them and I wanted to know them also. There was an operational definition of love for me. I wanted to kiss them, praise them, listen to them, treasure their curiosity, play with them in a gentle way, encourage their intellect and laugh together.

That was the purpose of our early morning conversations and checker games. There was a dosage of stories of Jeff as an eight year old boy and laughter as Alison told me about some of her friends and likes and thoughts. I shared some of my likes with her. I told her about the stickball and basketball games Jeff and I played nearly every Saturday and Sunday for years, except when Jeff had Little League games.

We took a walk or two along the narrow shore line before noon as the rest of the group talked and read by the blanket and the beach chairs. Sometimes she and I held hands as we walked and talked and sometimes she walked alone. Alison picked up clamshells, small white and colored stones and once she saw a skate, one that was devoured by seagulls.

There were two significant events that happened once we arrived at Long Beach Island and the house we rented. They were so subtle that I suspect I didn't understand the significant of them until it was time for me to go home from the vacation. No one worried about my comings and goings when I took my daily walks and I surely didn't. The other tactful change that happened was that Anne and Jeff trusted me to baby-sit for Alison and Jessica when Anne and Jeff worked out. It was subtle but it was significant to me. It showed me that I was able to care for my granddaughters and that Anne and Jeff knew that and trusted me and I knew that they wouldn't say it if it wasn't true. They wouldn't compromise their daughters' safety at all.

When we first got to Long Beach Island I looked around the block where our rental house was so that I could find some landmarks, a unique house or a fence or store or big hedge, to help make my way back to the house after I took a walk daily. There were street signs but I wasn't sure that I could remember the name of the street on which we lived; thus the landmarks. I walked the flat streets everyday alone at about 8 or 8:30 a.m. for about three or four miles. That took me somewhere about 45 to 110 minutes. People on Long Beach Island were exercise freaks but nice friendly polite exercise freaks. My kind of people. Walkers, runners and even some bike riders and some people who sat on the porches said "Hi" as they passed me by or I passed them. All I had to do was say "Hi" back and smile a polite smile back to them. I perfected the "Hi" and smile and I enjoyed my morning walks because of the "Hi" and the smile.

By the time I got back to the house Dale, Anne and Jeff were up and around. Dale just started her walk. Either Anne or Jeff walked. The other one watched Alison and Jessica.

Once I came home the other one lit out for an early morning jog also. I watched television with Alison and Jessica. It was a grandpa's joy. I was enchanted by the hypnotic spell that the Disney channel had on them. For a second or two the spell was broken and we talked and almost in a split second they again had that focused look in their eyes. Again the spell was broke and they asked for a bagel or some more cereal or a piece of toast or juice or milk.

By eleven we were on the sandy beach and the glimmering ocean called out to me to swim. I was a pretty good swimmer not just when I was a kid in high school but in my fifties. I participated in three triathlons and though I finished last in all of them, I was proud of it. I did in fact do well in the first part of the race which was the mile swim and I was in the middle of the pack when I came out of the ocean for the bike ride. So I wasn't chopped liver either. Anyway I walked to the water and touched my toes in. Slowly I did an old man's walk in. I did that walk from the time I was a lifeguard in Coney Island. Once the water reached my waist I dove in and swam a couple of butterfly strokes. I had that feeling of carefree exuberance, the strength of my arms and shoulders, the cool water on my face, the speed of my body as I glided through the little waves, that was the sensation that I felt, and the excitement of bodysurfing back to the beach. And the best part of it was that no one made a big deal about the "fragile" nature of my health. On the contrary, Dale, Jeff and Anne laughed and said that I looked good and Jeff smiled when he marveled about my high freestyle strokes in the water. I was a good ocean swimmer, but I knew that I wasn't a legend in my mind ever, not even a contender, not even a contender to be a contender. The rest of the week was terrific. Jeff and I and sometimes Dale went bodysurfing for as much as an hour. Jeff spent some time boogie boarding while I bodysurfed.

Anne and Jeff got some time in the water when Dale and I sat with Jessica. Alison was a big girl, she was four and half years old so she didn't need us as babysitters, but she kept us company and she read her own books. She was a great reader and she took walks with Dale and me. Sometimes it was with just Dale and once in awhile with just me. But it was clear from the moment that she walked on the sand that she was a beach person. She had her books, her sunglasses, her chair, her sunscreen, her water bottles, her sandwiches, and her interest in sea creatures and shells. Her persona screamed beach person as she walked with Anne and Dale. Although Alison was reluctant to go into the ocean for the first couple of days she came around. By the last day on the beach she loved to have Dale and I swing her over the waves. Her laughter is still heard in my memory so that when I need it today I can retrieve it and smile to myself.

We spent most of our time on the beach blanket and chairs. Anne watched Jessica underneath the blue and white umbrella that Jeff screwed into the sand to shade Jessica. Anne did spend time on the porch so that Jessica could sleep in a cool room. As I remember Jeff, Dale and I helped out a little also. We allowed Anne to get to the beach as we babysat for Jessica. The point was that I did have a role in this family vacation and I suspect the role was not diminished by my stroke and for that I loved Jeff and Anne. But Jessica's presence was evident at once when she came to the blanket. There was the cooing, the conversations, the effect of two children on Anne and Jeff, the bottles and food she ate, her clothing size and the small pool that was filled up with salt water, shovels, pails and balls.

Sure I talked and I was part of the conversations that took place but I wasn't the center of the conversations nor should I and that was one of the best lessons for me. I listened and took measure of the thoughts, but one thought at a time, and laughed at jokes and witticisms. Alison read also and she listened to the conversations and periodically she wanted an explanation or two. It was Anne who looked very relaxed, happy and content. I enjoyed the give and take with Anne and Jeff.

There were hodgepodges of events that rounded out our vacation at Long Beach Island. There were luncheonettes which had great scrumptious breakfasts. We ate in three of them and they all were kid friendly. We ate in restaurants for four dinners. The first day in Long Beach Island, Beach Haven, New Jersey, we ate at the Boathouse. We brought in a case of beer and two bottles of wine. We ordered appetizers, tostados with guacamole, salsa, and olives, and clams and shrimp and grilled calamari. The entrees were mouthwatering tequila mahi-mahi, tuna, jumbo crab cakes and orange ginger glazed salmon. Alison ate fish fries or hotdogs or hamburgers. She had wonderful manners when we ate. It was a joy to be with her and I was very proud of her. I was able to give my own orders to the waitresses most of the time. Once in awhile Dale shot out the end of my order and I was upset with myself and her for a second or two but I was thrilled to be there and I wasn't going to screw it up. We ate dinner at the rental house two or three times and it was a feast. Jeff and I had a dozen clams. We all had shrimp and salads as appetizers. There were two entrées that we ate. One, we got from the Shack Rack, it included the most delicious BBQ Spare Ribs, Chicken and French fries smothered with BBQ sauce. And the other one we got from M&M Seafood Market. We got five crab cakes and three one and a half pound lobsters with butter. Jeff made up a batch of margaritas for the appetizers. There were margaritas, beer and wine to accompany the entrée.

There were two major changes for me when I ate. I reduced significantly my intake of food especially when I went to Long Beach Island. I ate no more than two BBQ Spare Ribs, less than a quarter of a chicken breast, four or ten French fries, and lobster with lemon but with no butter. After we ate we went out for a large yogurt sugar cone.

I ate those kinds of food once a year for a week and one meal at Katz's and one meal for Passover. The rest of the year I limited my salt intake to no more than 1000 mg daily. I ate organic whole grains cereal for breakfast with orange juice and an apple almost daily. I ate either a low sodium turkey sandwich with mustard or a can or two of tuna in water with some balsamic vinegar and maybe a sweet onion and an apple or an orange. Dinner was made by Dale. We ate skinless chicken breast with vegetables and either a baked potato or brown rice, or salmon with vegetables and brown rice, or pasta dish, or a rack of lamb with vegetables and brown rice. I limited the number of alcoholic drinks that I drank to no more than one bottle of beer or one glass of merlot or two glasses of sangria. I drank merlot most of time.

There were many wonderful moments at Long Beach Island. The most precious was the love and security I felt from Dale, Jeff, Anne, and Alison and I thought even Jessica. I still was aware of my speech/language handicaps. It was still not feasible for me to follow more than one conversation or more than one person talking at a time. I surely couldn't deal with a barrage of staccato questions and answers. But the joy exceeded anything that I imagined. I remembered that I thought about the unparalleled ecstasy of these moments. I felt blessed and I was not a religious person. I understood the joy at the time it happened and that happened infrequently in the past. There was a lesson if and only if I could remember daily that I was alive and glad to be alive and there were more joyful moments in my life in my future if I allowed them to come in to my life.

Predators

There were people who were cruel, nasty, sadistic and insidious. They were few and far between and they were mostly unknown to me, impersonal, and quickly forgotten. At the most they warrant a mental quiet "fuck you" or a finger. There was one and only one person out of about forty people in my extended family who tried to humiliate me in public, laughing about my speech, my difficulties finding words, and later in my home.

It was about five years ago and life moved on. My wife and I denounced those actions by the person in front of others and I spoke about it with Peggy and Pierre. Everything was made transparent, the person was unmasked. I wasn't able to hold in my rage. Words came out forcibly, stuttering, faltering, and incoherently. My arms went back and forth because I couldn't control them when I was upset. It was as if I was back to my day's right after my stroke.

There was no reason to dwell on this anymore. There was a lukewarm apology. It had no meaning to me. Only action will have meaning to me in the future. It was meant to placate me and my wife. Ultimately, we just wanted everything to be civil, calm and reasonable. And so I accepted it because it allowed us to share holidays, birthdays, births, school graduations, and other important dates for extended family members.

I wanted you, the reader, to understand, feel, the depth of the insults and degradation. But spirit decontamination by definition is done alone. It is the purification of body and mind for rape victims, the long showers meant to scrub every pore so that the mind can get some peace, nights of nightmares, and days of resentment. Peggy and my friend Pierre allowed me to talk virtually daily about those insults to me so that I could erase away the stench of these terrible memories.

It will and does pass. The memories linger like a sinkhole, sometimes it stinks more than other times. But these are in truth only moments, limited moments. What I needed to do was to keep my eyes on the ball and that ball was "huge grandpa huge grandpa", that was Alison's expression. With all the joy I have in my life I don't really care about one person's flaw as long as I don't have to feel, see or hear it anymore.

September 2002 - Reestablishment of My Consultancy in Middletown, New York

September 2002 was significant for me. I started a new contract for two elementary and two middle schools with the Middletown School District. I had all the skills that I needed to complete my tasks. I was able to enter data very slowly, make very simple data analysis, use a boilerplate to write formative reports and discuss the programs with all four principals for English language arts and mathematics. Most of the principals made it clear to me that they understood my ideas, concepts and principles. It took a little more time but the results were worthwhile from their point of view. In some cases they improved student scores by about 10 percentage points on state tests.

I was asked to participate in two or three meetings with the Assistant Superintendent, a few of Directors and a couple of Coordinators after school. The Assistant Superintendent asked me an open question about the delivery of instruction in fourth grade and eighth grade English language arts or mathematics. I remember the huge pit in my stomach as I tried to formulate my answers and wing answers that should have been a piece of cake at least before my stroke. Unfortunately, I couldn't even outline an answer in my head. I couldn't remember the words in the question and I couldn't find words that I needed to use to explain my thoughts. Yet there were enough words that were part of my fabric, words that I used daily for nearly fifteen years. These words helped me to structure some phrases or sentences. Sometimes I just couldn't find the words. These high priced administrators, some of whom were empathetic, some of whom were embarrassed for me and that was unnecessary, and some who were annoyed to have to sit at a meeting with me and listen to my limited vocabulary, got the meat of my thoughts clearly. It wasn't pretty but they understood the gaps in the various programs. They understood the concerns about the scope and sequence of each program. It took a lot of energy out of me.

As I drove to the Holiday Inn I marveled about my vigor through all these years and my need to now conserve this power. I smiled to myself, not a smile of tricky but an inner smile because of my chutzpah. If necessity is the mother of invention than my love for my sons fathered the muscle in part to overcome the handicaps from my stroke. I was proud of myself.

To conserve my energy I worked smart and efficiently. Rather than driving 100 miles back and forth daily for three days bimonthly. I went up early on Tuesday. I took the Long Island Railroad at 7 a.m. to Penn Station. From Penn Station I took the Path to Hoboken, New Jersey. At Hoboken I took the Metro North train to Middletown. I arrived somewhere at 11-12. I slept on the Metro North train for about 45 minutes. I read a couple of pages in a book. Dale packed me a sandwich, a bottle of orange juice, water and a trail mix conglomeration made of almonds, grapes, Sun-Maid Golden Raisins, and an apple or bananas or orange.

Once I got to Middletown, Enterprise took me to their office and gave me a rental car for two or three days. This allowed me to drive from school to school and meeting to meeting. It permitted me to control my time better than if I used taxis. I was able to go to a school at a specific time, get some lunch away from the school, get a twenty minute nap or so and go to another school. I was able to buy some fruit and a bottle of Poland Spring water at the Middletown Shop and Stop. Across from the Shop and Stop was a liquor store. I was able to buy three splits of merlot. Every night I drank a glass of wine. Enterprise took me back to the train when it was time for me to go home, that was at about 3:10 p.m.

I went to the Holiday Inn for two days. I ate breakfast and dinner most of the time at the Holiday Inn. By the time I finished work I got to the Holiday Inn at about 4:30p.m., drank a bottle of water, put on the television and took a nap for about an hour. Later, I ate and drank a glass of merlot

and I put the television on. At about 8:30 I worked
about two hours and took my medicine. Dale put
medicine in two separate different seven day medi
boxes, one for morning pills and one for evening pi
read a page or two in a book, and then I went to sleep.
was a more restful day than I would have had should I
driven home daily.

To make sure that I was healthy I made an appointment
with a cardiologist in Middletown prior to my bimonthly
trips to Middletown. I wanted to make sure that there was a
specific cardiologist in Middletown who knew my medical
condition should I have another heart attack or a stroke. I
made sure that I put his name, address and telephone
number in my daily reminder weekly calendar. I saw the
cardiologist twice. It made me feel more secure when I
traveled to Middletown and went about my business.

October 2002 Progress Report

Peggy wrote a progress report on me for the period from
August, September, and October 2002. She indicated that I
complained about my difficulties with my auditory memory
for details, my inability to access my "fund of knowledge"
because I couldn't synthesize and analyze information at
my normal speed and precision, and my inability to
"follow" conversations with several people with my former
pace and sharpness intact. My writing skills improved. I
was able to compose personal letters and e-mails. I wrote
daily and improved my syntactical and semantic skills yet
when Peggy tested me on October 24, 2002 I demonstrated
ambiguous word choices and errors on articles (a, the,
there) and prepositions. Peggy wrote down that my
expressive language skills were found to be "mildly",
"moderately" and or "impaired" and characterized by
difficulty with verbal fluency, verbal specificity, writing
skills (e.g. speed, semantics), circumlocution, eye contact,
vocal intensity, and speed of processing.

After October 24 Peggy noted that she worked with me to address areas of weakness that were demonstrated on the neuropsychological examination, including auditory memory and speed on tasks. Peggy observed that I scored 50% on a written direction task and 60% on recall of facts from a paragraph. She pointed out that in more recent sessions I improved my scores to 100% and 75% respectively. In the progress report Peggy characterized my going back to my consulting work as "initially overwhelming" and pointed out that I demonstrated halted speech due to persisting aphasia. In the summary of the progress report Peggy noted my motivation was appropriate and consistent and highlighted "Difficulty continues with auditory recall, following 2-3 step directive, difficulty with higher level communication tasks, (e.g. inferential and abstract skills), verbal fluency and specificity and consistent use of compensatory strategies."

Peggy recommended that I get speech therapy three times a week for one hour a day. Her short term goals for me were to improve:

◊ auditory recall at complex sentence level of names, dates, time to 90% over 20 trials,
◊ following 2-3 step verbal directives to 80% over 10 trials,
◊ inferential (abstract thinking) skills to 90% over 10 trials,
◊ verbal fluency and specificity to 90% over 15 trials,
◊ use of compensatory strategies given min/mod cues to improve receptive/expressive skills to WNL,
◊ speed of processing on written tasks when writing 3-4 paragraph length material,
◊ ability to identify and self correct errors in written work, and
◊ ability to describe complex pictures in a timely manner with increased specificity

Somewhere between August and October 2002 I read two books, Bernard Lewis's <u>What Went Wrong</u> and Franz Kafka's <u>The Metamorphosis and Other Stories</u>. I had started the Lewis book just before my stroke on February 2002. It had been a best seller and I also heard about the book on television although I don't know whether it was on the news or it was on a Charlie Rose program or Brian Lamb's <u>C-Span</u> program.

By the time I actually read the book it was nearly ten months after my stroke. It was a must read book. I wanted to understand more than the cursory views of the political, social, economic, scientific changes in the Middle East shown on television or written in the articles found in the <u>New York Times.</u> I wanted to understand the disconnection between the Muslim world and Christendom. I read the book while the United States of America took revenge on Afghanistan, Al Qaeda and Osama bin Laden for the brutal wanton murder of my countrymen. But I don't remember whether the Bush administration unleashed their public relations bomb on my countrymen, Europe and the United Nations and the lies of Weapons of Mass Destruction.

But I do know that I read this tiny book daily until I finished it. It wasn't just for the theoretical information. It wasn't for the abstract. It was for concrete words, changes and behaviors even though I didn't know what those explicit words, changes and behaviors would be. It was also important for me to relearn words such as "Ottoman Empire", "caliphate", and "slavery". As I remember this period of my recovery these words unleashed a multitude of other words and thoughts. Once I was able to pronounce the "Ottoman Empire" there surged other words and events. There was a free flow of words, events and ideas, such as "Russia", "Czar", "Russian Revolution", "Lenin", "Trotsky", "socialists", "World War I", "Triple Alliance", "Austria Hungarian Empire", "Metternich", "Germany", "Kiser", "England", "Lloyd George", "France",

"Clemenceau", "Woodrow Wilson" and "Versailles Treaty". There were many secondary words, events and people. The problem was that I couldn't necessarily repeat all the words, events and ideas again but I was able to remember some and forget others. Unfortunately, I couldn't spell all of these words in my head or on paper.

The words "caliphate" and "slavery" triggered off a free flow of more words and issues. It was very difficult for me to pronounce "caliphate". I knew the word in my mind. I could feel it. I knew that I knew it from my Latin American studies, but I couldn't get the word out from my mind. I tried to pronounce it. I couldn't and I tried again and again. Finely, when I started to read another couple of words the word "caliphate" came out of my mouth, a couple of times and then I couldn't pronounce it again. The next day when I got up I said at once "Caliphate of Cordova". I repeated that maybe ten times. It triggered a free flow of more words and issues. There were words such as "crusades", "Christians", "Muslims", "Jews", "Spain", "Portugal", "Pope", "Isabel and Fernando", "Columbus", and "Indians".

This was true for "slavery" also. "Slavery" had different legal, social and religious implications for slaves in Biblical and Greek times, the essence of their humanity and their manumission. It had different legal, social and religious implications for Catholics and Protestants in the colonies, in the United States of America and Brazil. Lewis pointed out the religious nuances in the Muslim world for slaves. It triggered a free flow of more words and issues. But the most important thing for me was my ability to synthesize thoughts and ideas. It was so exciting to me, my ability to read words, understand ideas, analyze thoughts and synthesize principles and concepts. It was a first. It was a rush. It was a first step for me but a very powerful rush nevertheless.

My reading Franz Kafka's The Metamorphosis and Other Stories had a different ring for me. It was a classic. If I read other classics, as I did before my stroke, than it was not significant for me to read a specific book, after all I read hundreds of books many of them were classics. But after I had my stroke and I couldn't read, speak or write it was very important to me, once I could read, even in a limited way, to read a classic as soon as I could. This 191 page book was on my bed stand, or on the kitchen table or living room table, it was where I was. Once when I thought about it I smiled to myself. It reminded me of a student who lugs heavy books, weighty books, known books, classic books so that other students and teachers would know that he was a serious student. I remembered graduate students, teachers and administrators who did the same.

Every day at dinner I told Dale about Franz Kafka's The Metamorphosis and Other Stories. I suspect that I did this to reinforce my own belief that I really could read and read a book that was intellectually challenging, a classic. I know that I did this also to make sure that there were conversations as Dale and I ate supper. It made me a worthwhile husband and companion, someone who could share ideas and thoughts and laughter. It was the passageway for Dale and me to talk with each other. It allowed me to listen to Dale's ideas and thoughts and laughter. I enjoyed the tangents that came out of these discussions. My stuttering was not really important to Dale once my thoughts coalesced. Dale got the main ideas and most of the details of my part of our conversations. There was laughter and disagreement about ideas and thoughts. There was tranquilly and anger about interpretations. There was contentment and frustration on fundamental principles and concepts. But in the main, day in and day out, I thought that there was life for Dale and me, our, I, me, had a brain and we shared our brains with each other, that was sexy for me.

There was another reason for my reading Franz Kafka's The Metamorphosis and Other Stories. I wanted to become a writer, not an author of only education books and articles but nonfiction and fiction books that have a soul and spirit, with words that sing out a message in breathtaking words. I

119

wanted to learn the way words and phrases were used to write classics. Every day I read Franz Kafka's The Metamorphosis and Other Stories aloud, word by word, phrase by phrase, sentence by sentence, paragraph by paragraph, and page by page.

Most of the time I was able to read whole words, but I was not able to fuse words together fluently. When I read aloud my words were choppy. They didn't flow. Every word was a sentence. But the fact that I was able to read whole words meant that I continued to grow. I would feel it, and that excited me.

What was more exciting was that these words opened the floodgates of my dreams, dreams that I never shared before my stroke and now my goals were focused. It was ironic that it took my stroke to make me fully aware of my feelings, more observant and more disciplined to reach my goal. I once heard someone say that if you get up in the morning and you write and you write and you do that daily you are a writer. I was a writer. Imagine that, ten months after my stroke, there was a metamorphosis. I started as a stroke victim and I grew into a writer.

Relearning to Write

From the first day I entered into Transitions of Long Island I had to write, admittedly, in the most cursory manner. I had to try to copy my first and last name, the date, day and period of each class that I took daily. It was difficult for me. I couldn't spell the words. I had to look at the blackboard after each letter not word but letter. Within a week or two I was able to write my name, I don't know whether I wrote my name accurately right away. I had to write my homework assignments. Again I copied it from the blackboard letter by letter. When I started to work with Deena and especially Peggy they told me my assignments and either told me the letters in each word or wrote the assignment for me.

Somewhere in late spring early summer 2002 Peggy asked me to copy and write some sentences and later paragraphs and letters. I copied sentences from the <u>New York Times</u> and from articles written by Ms. Dowd and Mr. Rich. The earliest sentences and smallest paragraphs were for the most part political. This was a sample of what I did.

1. In Cairo, President Mubarck said that Egyptian intelligence officials warned American intelligence officials about Osama bin Laden's plan to target American sites. Although CIA senior officials denied that Egyptian intelligence discovered the plots there were sign that they were escalations. Congress needs to know if President Mubarck was truthful and if the CIA and FBI were honest. The September 11 tragically needs to investigate.

2. In the aftermath of September 11, Congressional committees differ such as the Senate Judiciary committee and joint oversight committee. Some of them favor more freewheeling and aggressive investigation. Others are too close to the F.B.I. and C.I.A. Representative Goss of the joint oversight committee was a C.I.A. officer. Another problem for investigators is the finger pointing of C.I.A. and F.B.I.

3. Maureen Dowd, editorial/op-ed reporter, shows the tragicomedy played out by the F.B.I and C.I.A. after September 11, 2002. The C.I.A.-F.B.I rivalry, known as the Wedge, was part of the religion-economic culture clash between Catholic Fordham and Notre Dame and WASP Ivy Princeton and Harvard. However, the cliché is totally flipped at the top. Mr. Tenet, C.I.A. director, is the son of Greek immigrants while Mr. Mueller, F.B.I director, is a Princeton graduate. These agencies continue there "circling the wagons" and harm our country. F.B.I. blames the C.I.A. and the C.I.A. blames the F.B.I. And Al Qaeda laughs.

4. The horrific deaths cause by Al Qaeda and Osama bin Laden of September 11 was tragic. Al Qaeda

and Osama bin Laden were murders. They caused carnage and destroyed innocent lives. These fanatical Islamic zealots annihilated over 3,000 people in New York City and Virginia.

5. But there was another tragedy. There was a conspiracy by the President, Vice President, military officials, and corporations. These were provocateurs. These "American leaders" saw an opportunity to capitalize on these Islamic zealots. They knew about the general plans of Osama bin Laden and seized their moment. In one flash, Mr. Bush and his entire right wing Republican Christian coalition, they became our America. Mr. Bush changed from a minority president into the President. Any American who challenged Mr. Bush's policies was labeled "unpatriotic" by Mr. Vice President Cheney. Our military increased and our young women and men were troops for Christendom. They were doing battle against evil. In one flash, our economy improved. More arms, ships, and weapons. There was no social security problem, no welfare problem, and no medical problem.

Unfortunately, I didn't save each sentence and paragraph as I wrote them. I did save them in my computer file, that file condensed many weeks if not months of writing. I'm not able to state accurately whether paragraph 1 was written in one day or did it take a couple of days to complete the next sentence and another couple of days for another couple of sentences. Also, I'm not sure whether Dale just looked at my homework or proofed it. My best recollection was that she just looked at it. I understood that my homework was my homework not Dale's. I knew that I had to put great energy into my writing if I wanted to be made "whole" and to write letters, articles, reports and books. It was important for me to work through my writing problems and those problems were in my brain also. That stroke of mind had many hidden physical, neurological and psychiatric manifestations. One of them was writing.

From February to April 2002 I was not able to write original sentence. By late spring, I was able to copy couple of sentences from an article and write them out. That meant that I was able to read the sentences, understand them, copy each letter and word letter by letter and word by word until the sentences were printed out from my printer. There wasn't an original word or thought in those print outs. By the middle of the summer, I copied two sentences and make them into one sentence more or less. That meant that I was able to read the sentences, understand them, copy each letter and word letter by letter and word by word and put in a preposition "and", "but" and "yet" that made two sentences into one. Again, except for the prepositions, there were no original words or thoughts in the print out. By the end of the summer, or early fall, I was able to summarize the essence of a very small article and write a little paragraph with many original words and thoughts and concepts such as Paragraph 5. That meant that I was able to read the sentences, understand them, copy each letter and word letter by letter and word by word, put in a preposition "and", "but" and "yet" that made two sentences into one, and write original words and thoughts and concepts. I had to give great thought about a word or thought or concept. It wasn't that I had to try to write down the letters and words. It was more than that.

Unfortunately, even today, I couldn't spell words correctly. In most cases I couldn't remember the words for my thoughts once I had had my thoughts. When my words and thoughts stuck in my brain I still had the problem of how to form the words letter by letter. I couldn't figure out the first letter of the word and the second and third letter also but that first letter of a word was a killer. I didn't know whether the word started with a "t" or a "d" or a "b" or a "p". I couldn't separate the "n" from an "m". Even when I knew a word in my brain that wasn't a sure bet that I could spell the word. I was a daunting task to figure out a word and spell it.

ı ortunately, my computer and Microsoft Word helped me. At the top of the page in Microsoft Word, horizontally, were nine words starting at the left side of the page with "File" and ending with "Help". The sixth word from the left side of the page was "Tools". I click open "Tools". The drop screen for "Tools" included "Language". "Language" included "Thesaurus". "Thesaurus" provided me with the correct spelling of a word, a list of synonyms and antonyms and identified the parts of speech. To use the "Thesaurus" I had to write down the word in a Microsoft Word file. Once I wrote the word and clicked once on the word and then took my mouse pointer to "Tools", "Language" and "Thesaurus" I would know whether the word was spelled correctly or not. In some cases, if there were enough correct letters in a word, the program corrected the word. If not I worked hard to find the correct letters in a word until the "Thesaurus" decided that I gave it enough information to find the word. For example, if I wanted to write the word "vociferous" and I wrote it as "vorcifers" the "Thesaurus" would not show the word "vociferous", but if I wrote the word "vociferus" it would come up as "vociferous" and there would be eight synonyms and one antonym.

Given my limited vocabulary and my inability to spell well at this time I used the "Thesaurus" for most of my writing. That meant that most of my time was spent in looking up words in the "Thesaurus". It was tedious but it helped me to improve my spelling. After I verified a word I always looked as the lists of synonyms and antonyms and identified the parts of speech. Each word helped me to learn others. I still have to use this strategy to write. I still needed to use the "Thesaurus".

Without my laptop computer, a gift from Jeff, Anne, and Alison a year before my stroke for my birthday and father's day, I would have not made the gains that I had in writing. When I first used my laptop after my stroke I had to relearn the keyboard. Each time that I tried to write a word I used the "Thesaurus". Peggy pushed me to use my computer. She wanted me to e-mail her my homework. At that time I wasn't willing to do that. It would have taken too much energy to write any e-mails, write the message, correct the words, and format the e-mail, and acknowledge to myself everyday that I was a functional illiterate. I knew it. Peggy knew it. And yet I didn't want Peggy to know the intensity that I had to put in to an e-mail. I worked on a two or three sentences e-mail for two days before I sent the e-mail to Peggy. It was one homework assignment. That was my craziness, my vanity.

Peggy pushed me hard in different ways, she bore down on my writing, she pressed me to remember history and she compelled me to explain my thoughts to her from my writings. One of the first assignments that Peggy gave me was on the Bible. The homework had five questions. Peggy gave me The Dictionary of Cultural Literacy for my birthday. She wrote in the book that my "motivation, determination and courage are testimony to your boldness in facing adversity as you strive towards regaining the power of communication!" It was a very thoughtful gift. I would say the same thing to her and all the people who do her work. It must be one of the most difficult professions and Peggy's motivation, determination and courage helped me to be a life. Peggy, thank you.

This was the homework that Peggy gave me. It took me four or five days to finish this assignment. I read 27 pages in The Dictionary of Cultural Literacy about the Bible, most of my energy was not focused on the New Testament not because of Jesus and Christianity but because the questions were mostly on the Old Testament. There was a stirring as I read the 27 pages, organized the events, people and issues and wrote my answers. Most of the words that I needed and used were found in the book but I used them in different ways. And some words were not found at all. Those words were me. All the tedious and exasperating work that went into the preparation for writing the assignment disappeared the second that I wrote my first original sentence and paragraph. No copying a sentence verbatim. No. No. No. Paragraphs 3, 4 and 5 paraphrased and synthesized information from the book and I made my answers my answers. It was my thoughts and me, just me and my "Thesaurus".

BIBLE

1. The Bible is the basis for Judaism and Christianity.
2. In the Bible, Judaism and Christianity cite Adam and Eve as the first people.
3. In the Bible, Judaism and Christianity believe that God is the alpha and omega from Adam and Eve to the angels, final apocalypse and Armageddon and the Messiah.
4. There are two Bibles. Jews and Christians believe in the 39 books of the Old Testament while only the Christians being in the 27 books of the New Testament. There are different lessons in the Bible. On one side God is just. Those are the stories of Adam and Eve, Tower of Babel, Cain and Abel and Jacob and Joseph, Judas Iscariot and Pontus Pilate. On the other side God is merciful. Those are the accounts of the Book of Genesis and the Book of Exodus. Those are the covenants of Noah, Abraham and Moses. There is the burning bush when God is revealed to Moses, or the Sermon of the Mount and the prayer that Blessed are the peacemakers and the crucifixion of Jesus and Jesus' words "Father, Forgive Them For They From Not What They Did".
5. The Bible is both a moral creed and a description of human frailties. From the beginning, the Bible clarified ethical, just, righteous, and virtuous traits. These included the Fall of Man, the Mosaic Law and Yom Kippur, the Golden Rule, the Book of Exodus and the Ten Commandant. On the other side there were stories of human problems. These were the accounts of David and Goliath, Esther, Mordecai and Puriom (sic), and Elajah (sic) and Jezebel.

As I finished one homework assignment Peggy gave me another assignment. I don't know the sequence exactly of these assignments. They were about the same time, no more than a week away, somewhere six months after my stroke. This task dealt with Idioms. Peggy gave me nine idioms and I had to write a sentence or two for each. It was a frustrating assignment but by the time I fulfilled it it showed me that I moved up to another intellectual level. These required me to read words, understand idioms, find words in my brain, spell words, and write a simple sentence. It was arduous for me to search my brain and find the appropriate words to define the idiom. Once I found the word or words it was laborious to spell it, most of the time I had to use the "Thesaurus". By the time I finished it I was spent. Yet there was a rush, the excitement of writing original sentences, the ability to find the appropriate words, spell them and write a legible sentence. These were my sentences.

IDIOMS
1. According to Hoyle- A person has to follow rules
2. Ace in the hole-Sometimes you need to have an trick up your sleeve
3. Achilles' heel-In many instances even the "best" people limitations or weaknesses
4. Act of God-There is not any reasonability for what happens to some people
5. Ad absurdum- Faculties go to lengths to prove hypoteses are ridiculous
6. Life of Riley- Now that I am a senior citizen I live the life of Riley.
7. Make a mountain out of a molehill-Sometimes I am not sure that a person's rude behavior warrants my making a mountain out of a molehill.
8. Nose out of joint-I am upset by mischievous behavior and that causes my nose out of joint.
9. Pay the piper-Because of my stroke and my speech some "members" of my extended family want to make me pay the piper.

Writing was a solitary exercise and my thoughts and my writing style were uniquely mine too. At this point I didn't have a real handle on my thoughts and I surely didn't have any writing style but what I had was me. It was my

127

thoughts and my style. It wasn't Dale's, Jeff's, Anne's or Pierre's. It was mine. Each word that I put on paper, each original sentence that I wrote, as simple as it was, was me. My writing, as limited as it was, it was me. Each sentence that I wrote was sacramental. It went to my core, racked my brain, shook my confidence and was an outer feeling of my inner thoughts, fears and hopes.

There was a symbiotic relation, the more I wrote the more I had control of my life and the more I had control of my life the more I wrote. Peggy, Dale, Jeff, Anne and Pierre were cheerleaders, each in different ways. They dealt with me with gentility, never roughly. They prodded and cajoled me. They remembered with me. They listened to my writings. They encouraged me. And they believed me when I said that I would write an article or book about my stroke.

The truth be told I didn't know that I could really write an article much less a book until each of them told me that that was a great idea, no doubts on their parts, no doubts that I could. That was strong spiritual encouragement. It was the fiber that made me think that I might be able to write an article or book. When I put out a trial balloon, Robert and Erick automatically thought that it was a done deal after all if I said that I would write an article or book than I would write an article or book, no big deal. They don't know how much that meant to me. They believed that I could do what I said so I believed it too. They made me think that I could be a writer. When Pierre told me that he would edit any manuscript that I wrote I knew that this was real. It wasn't just a pie in the sky dream. In a split second I had my verification that I was a writer. I would write about my stroke. Ultimately, the support that I got from family and friends helped me to write this book. Each day I wrote a page I felt suitable to the task, and that gave me more control of my life.

Relearning to Sing

When the dust cleared from my eyes and the grime from my soul when the corridors of <u>Transitions of Long Island</u> were seen not as empty halls but areas of friendly conversations and communications with concerns, smiles and laughter, when unknown people were turned into recognized acquaintances, then and only then was I able to make music important to me again and that was in the summer of 2002.

Music was part of my daily life from the time I was a kid to the day I had my stroke. As a kid I loved Yiddish music on the radio. I still love hearing Romania, Romania. Most of the music from 1940's -1980's came from <u>It's The Make Believe Ballroom</u>. Today that music is classified as "elevator music". To me it was a conglomeration of Frank Sinatra, Bing Crosby, Rosemarie Clooney, The Gershwin's, Ella Fitzgerald, Johnnie Mathis, and Perry Como. It was the William B. William radio show. I liked Gospel, Blues, Jazz, Western, Folk, and Classical music also. I loved to hear the sounds of the Tango, the music of Argentina, sex and passion. My taste in music was eclectic. In other words it was music, music, music. I liked music, I liked music daily. I liked to hear it on my car radio and at the time of my stroke on my CDs and tapes in my car. There wasn't a day that I didn't sing to the music in my car. My car rides were sprinkled with my singing a duo with the likes of the Kingston Trio, Johnnie Cash, Chicago, Peggy Lee, Sinatra and Peter, Paul and Mary.

For at least six months I heard the music in my car but I was frustrated because I couldn't remember the words of the songs. I couldn't pronounce the words rapidly when I remembered some of the lyrics. I didn't know whether I would sing songs in my car ever. It felt damp, lonely and never ending the few times that I had to drive to Middletown, not because I drove slower but because it seemed to go on and on when I couldn't sing with the other artists in my car.

It was at this time that the majesty of <u>Transitions of Long Island</u> sparkled in ways that the bean counters in the insurance companies couldn't even fathom. One day as I was on my way out from Peggy's class I saw a bunch of people milling about on the second floor. Although I didn't know them I had seen them in the halls, stairs or elevators. I knew that they were out patients. One person told me that there was a sing-a-long. Anyone was invited. He gave me a flyer. There was the time and date. I sat down on chair and waited for about five minutes. All the people in the room spoke better than me. Their speech was fluent. Ultimately, there were about 15 people in the room. All of the people, except for me, were in classes together. They too had apraxia. The leader of the group, an out patient, handed out the lyrics for a song. I think it was a Joan Baez song Kumbaya.

It was great to sing again but I hesitated. I wasn't sure of the words and pronunciations. The group had a problem with the melody and the group leader stopped the group and walked us through both the words and the melody. I sang. Sometimes I couldn't get the words out of my mouth quickly and I flubbed parts of a line. But I sang. When we sang it over again I sang louder with greater confidence. It was a spiritual revival. In that room another part of my life was reconstructed. I knew that while I couldn't sing the complete song I knew that with time I could and would.

Today in 2006, each day I sing songs with a variety of artists. I'm not able to sing each song on the CDs or tapes or on the car radio, but I sing and I love to sing. Obviously, I'm more fluent in reading and speaking, but I'm still not perfect not even close. I flub a word, mispronounce a word, and forget the lyrics or melody. I don't remember most of the melodies and lyrics. I'm able to sing with the artists only when I hear the music on the CDs, tapes and radio. When I flub a word or line I go back and re-sing the song. I do that as much as five times in a row until I get it right. But that doesn't mean that I'll remember the lyrics and melody when I hear the CD the next day much less the next week. Yet I now sing parts and in some cases whole songs. The growth process continues to grow.

Conclusion

This chapter was about excitement, enjoyment, hope and more control and power over my life as I overcame significant limitations shown on my psychometric tests to my own self satisfaction. My own self observations showed me that I moved closer and closer to the person I was before my stroke.

I worked hard and I had a great group of supporters. I wanted to play a significant role in my granddaughters' lives so desperately and eventually I babysat for them and walked with them on the Long Beach Island beach and I beamed, oh I so beamed. I worked hard to participate in conversations with Dale, Jeff, Anne, Alison and Jessica during our vacation. It was wonderful when Jeff and I were able to laugh together. I wanted to become a more complete husband and I believed that the brain was one, if not the primary, sex organ so I read and discussed what I read with my wife. I worked hard to get my business back on track. There was the physical strain of traveling and the energy expended to explain ideas. But at the end of the day I felt proud on myself and I slept as only the content slept. That was true for music too as I worked hard to learn and sing songs. But it was true that each time I was able sing a song it brought a smile to my face. I worked hard to relearn to write. It was hard, monotonous, and lonely work but it was possible with a computer. When I saw the printer churn out words that I wrote and paraphrased words originally written by Maureen Dowd or Frank Rich it seemed to be a miracle too. I was able to get back my humanity and some of my control and power.

I appreciated what I had and I fought for my personal, civil and moral rights rather than always cursing God because I lacked something. I learned to dream all kinds of dreams.

Checklists

You need to:

◊   Remember, writing for a stroke survivor is very difficult. Think of a coal miner caught in a mine explosion. He can't see more than a foot or so. There are rocks all sizes that make it difficult if not impossible to know how to get out of his predicament. He doesn't know what he will find on the other side of a rock. He doesn't know if he can dig out from this. He doesn't know whether he has the strength to dig and he doesn't know whether there is enough air to keep him alive. This is a bird eye picture of a stroke survivor's brain trying to write the first time and he can't. Remember that writing is a slow, tedious and solitary process.

◊   Know the stages that you must go through to write:

1. Relearn your keyboard, learn to spell, and piece words into sentences.

2. Copy words, sentences and paragraphs

3. Make use of the spelling check and the thesaurus as you write your original sentences. Remember, you will spend most of your time trying to find the correct spelling for words.

4. Read your words aloud. Make sure they make sense in your sentence. Be wary about words such as "it", 'at" "an", "of", "or", and "to".

5. Write, write, write but allow yourself no more than two hours daily to write. Write letters write e-mails. Write to your congressmen and senator. The more you write the more control and power you will have.

6. Have your spouse, family member or friend edit your work daily.

◊ Listen to music daily. It is a great way to improve your conversational speech and the idioms used in American English.

◊ Go on a vacation with your spouse, family members or friends and participate in the conversations during meals and walks.

◊ Be like the little train that could, keep pushing and pushing, no matter what psychometric scores show just push and push each day every day. Equate reading, writing, listening, music and talking to people with sexiness, respect and pride.

Spouse and Friend need to:

◊ Encourage your spouse/friend to write. Be supportive and creative. Write an e-mail/letter from your office and ask family members, friends and acquaintances to do the same. Talk to your local school administrator and ask if one student could e-mail or send a letter to your spouse/friend.

◊ When your spouse/friend is comfortable edit his words/phrases/sentences. His thoughts are his thoughts. Don't put your thoughts or values as his. Just edit the words/phrases/sentences.

◊ If you want to have an enjoyable time once in awhile you might want to have a sing-a-long. It allows you and your stroke survivor to laugh, smile and kid around while it helps your spouse/friend to work on his/her memory, vocabulary, speech, and idioms.

◊ It is important to know that spouses/friends need to give back the power and control that was given to them by the stroke. It is an exceptional person who is sensitive enough to know when the stroke survivor is able to handle the power and control and relinquishes them.

Chapter 6: November 2002-May 2003
The Battle for My Dignity

Preview

This chapter deals with the last seven months of my rehabilitation as I was weaned from <u>Transitions of Long Island</u>. My whole world knew that I thought and existed. But I still had to struggle to reclaim my dignity, my essence, and who I was and my ability to love.

There were the customary activities. There were the monthly blood tests at the hospital. There were my medicines taken twice daily. There were the classes with Peggy. There was my work. There were my walks. There were my daily conversations with Dale. Anne and Jeff checked in nearly daily. There were the nearly daily talks with Pierre. These generated my self-respect daily.

There were the going and coming of friends and acquaintances a process that was necessary to grow maybe. Dale and I got together, every three or four weeks, with Anne, Jeff, Alison and Jessica. There were five birthdays from November to January and the holidays. There was the vacation in Puerto Rico, the sounds of Spanish, the beauty of the Island.

It was an intense period, an identifiable time, marked by major changes in the state of my mind and my relationships with family, and good friends. It was about privacy issues for me and my struggle to maintain any discretion on issues and events that related to just me. It was the cavalier way the insurance company limited my stay in therapy and the arrogant and abusive behavior of some police officers who knew little about the characteristics of stroke victims, aphasia and pacemakers and tried to undermine my dignity.

This chapter points out that all things stimulated my brain and my background knowledge helped me to defend myself and bolstered my dignity. Just being alive and seeing,

hearing, feeling and smelling strengthened my resolve. On a daily bases I could count on reading to allow me to feel a sense of pride. I spoke a couple of words in Spanish when Dale and I vacationed in Puerto Rico It was clear that I made gains but it was true that I had miles to go before I could take my place in the world that I left after my stroke and get my pre-stroke routine back and my dignity.
.

When you read this chapter you will be better prepared to:

◊ Enumerate what the word "dignity" means to you in real daily terms with real people and agencies.

◊ Deal with the mind numbing mentality of insurance companies and the weaning process from therapy.

◊ Share your expectations about the police, the way you want to be treated, and their knowledge of stroke and pacemaker survivors.

◊ Understand the multitude of ways to stimulate your mind, especially by reading, and thereby improve your self esteem.

◊ Acknowledge the singular blessing of family and friends.

My Progress Report November 2002 to January 2003

I continued receiving speech-language therapy three hours a week during one hour individual sessions at <u>Transitions of Long Island</u> from November 2002 to January 2003. At the end of that period Mrs. Kramer and Dr. Elbaum wrote a report on my progress, <u>This Report Constitutes Progress Report And Letter Of Medical Necessity For Ongoing Treatment For Donald Weinstein</u>. The report was based on my working with Peggy Kramer and on a speech-language re-evaluation performed on January 31, 2003. It made clear that I made some significant gains but I still had many miles to go.

There were gains in auditory memory, following oral directions, verbal fluency, providing synonyms and providing similarities and differences. I continued demonstrating significant gains in spontaneous conversation which included my ability to be interrupted and then return to the topic. I made gains in following 2-3 step verbal directives and improved my vocabulary and word retrieval ability. My integration of compensatory strategies had a positive effect on my overall receptive and expressive language scores. When I introduced a topic and held the speaker's role for a period of time my performance was good. With improvement in my semantic skills, verbal specificity improved moderately. In summary the report said that "Dr. Weinstein's motivation level and desire to attain maximal return to pre-stroke communication competence continues to be a driving force in his recovery, yet the effects of persisting aphasia preclude discharge at this time."

There were deficiencies, discrete problems for me from the period of October 24, 2002 to January 31, 2003. I had difficulty with auditory recall, particularly as the information becomes more lengthy and/or complex, or the speed of information presented is at a more 'normal' rate. I had difficulty with specific recall of details notwithstanding compensatory strategies. I didn't use these carryover strategies consistently. I didn't do well on inferential (abstract thinking) skills. The report said that I worked quickly on this sub-test and demonstrated a lack of attention to detail in the written material. Also, when challenged by more abstract tasks such as mental manipulation of the most basic level of numbers the true effects of my aphasia were frankly evident. My vocal tones become more subdued and my speed of processing was significantly slowed. My confidence level clearly diminished and paraphasic errors occurred. The report said I told Peggy that when a conversation was more quickly paced I lost my ability to follow resulting in frustration and self-consciousness. When in class I demonstrated delayed initiation, word retrieval, difficulty with thought organization and poor performance. On the other hand when I worked at home my writing ability improved significantly. The semantic and syntactic structures improved. My writing style expanded. I still hesitated due to word retrieval, particularly when given a specific task as opposed to spontaneous conversations. Sometimes I needed cues to be specific. For instance, when speaking about people, to provide their names or when relating a story on an incident, to slow my rate and better sequence events to more clearly make my point.

Birthdays and Holidays from
November to December 2002

My days were packed during the last two months of 2002. My consulting business was doing well. There were nearly daily talks with Pierre of God knows what. There were monthly blood tests for warfarin.

There were birthdays, holidays, religious and national holidays. There were birthdays for Alison (November 11), Lily (December 3), Erick (December 10) and Jessica (December 24). Erick was at Florida State University but there were parties for Alison and Jessica. Those were happy days and times. I never felt any stress when I went to Anne and Jeff's house for the parties for Alison and Jessica. Their birthdays were very special to me. It was joy for so many things. Only in my mind can I express the deep love, hope and worries that consumed me for them in this crazy world with so many quirks. Yet I would have momentary bursts of tears when I thought of Alison and Jessica and how I wanted them to have wonderful lives. My speech was as perfect as it could be with all the imperfections noted in the report written by Peggy at Transitions of Long Island.

The combined holidays of Thanksgiving Day and Christmas Day/Chanukah were always important to me but it meant more to me this year ten to eleven months after my stroke. I liked having all the extended family members over to our house. It was a chance for me to see all my sons and daughter-in-law and both of my granddaughters in one place. It made me happy for Dale. She saw her daughter and son-in-law, father, brother, and his significant friend, Stephanie and son Troy. Dale made tasty appetizers such as mushrooms, grilled kielbasa, shrimp, and salsa. Anne brought food as did Stephanie. The entrée was either delicious turkey with stuffing, potatoes and asparagus or beef burgundy. There was coffee, tea and dessert. Dale put on a great meal. There was non-ending banter, the hum of conversations, laughter, excitement, and the swap of gifts.

During this period of time there was a metamorphosis within me. I became aware that I enjoyed the conversations but I wasn't part of the conversations. Those couple of seconds that would have allowed me to be part of the discussions nearly never happened. By the time I wanted to put my two cents in, the conversation moved on. Most of the time there wasn't any eye contact with me. But there was a second or two when people scanned the faces of the other people in the group. It helped them to verify that the group got the point they made. Jeff, Anne and Dale made eye contact with me when they spoke with the group as did Stephanie. Stephanie always glanced at me when she said something to the group.

Sometime in this period I made up my mind that I would get back my personhood. Nobody would ignore me especially in my own home. I don't know when it happened and I know less about the process in my mind. I know that my daily conversations with Peggy, Dale, Jeff, Anne and Pierre made me more confident about my conversational speech. They understood me. But they were patient with me. I trusted my guests to be tolerant of me also. The easiest part for me was to say my sentence, with my stuttering and aphasia. There was some stress but not much. The stress came when they responded and asked me a question or made references to another part of the conversation that I forgot. These crossover conversations and staccato questions or answers were the bane of my mind. They were the reminder of how far I had to go to be part of my life again.

The process of reclaiming control and power of my life was evolutionary and yet revolutionary. Each step, driving, learning at Transitions of Long Island, working, going to the doctors by myself, writing checks, reading, writing, speaking, walking, exercising, traveling on trains, that I took from the first day at <u>Transitions of Long Island</u> was meant to help me, to take back my life and that had many implications to me but also to others. There were infinitesimal gains each day even though I couldn't see them through my eyes clearly. But Peggy did. Those minuscule improvements turned me into a grumpy, irritable, petulant, self centered, lovable, sometimes pain in the ass old man according to the people I most loved and respected.

Those who mocked me and tried to embarrass me in the past saw a proud unrelenting hardnosed man who would not take any more mistreatment, cruelty and insults from them. It made them crawl away in shame. I made sure that those who loved me understood clearly that the word "perception" was an insult to me. What I saw and felt was accurate, not a figment of my imagination, and they needed to understand that. I started to take back my control and power.

I Got a Pacemaker

On Sunday, December 1st, Dale took me to the emergency room and on December 3rd, I had a pacemaker put into me at <u>North Shore University Hospital</u>. I was referred for a pacemaker procedure because of Sinoatrial node dysfunction. I had a history of atrial fibrillation, conduction system disease and sick sinus syndrome. Dr. Matthew Fedor performed the surgery. He was the Chair of Electrophysiology Section of Division of Cardiology. I came home on Thursday December 5, 2002 and I went to class on Friday.

I think over the previous three or four months (September-November 2002) both Robert and Erick took me to the emergency room, I had felt faint. I have since learned that it was possible that my stroke could have been caused by my atrial fibrillation. It was possible that with medicine I could have avoided my stroke but I don't know. But "could have" and "should have" has no meaning to me now. It is what it is.

When I was at <u>North Shore University Hospital</u> Dale's son, Mark and his wife, Dana, had a little girl named Lily. I don't remember anything about that time. Dale told me that I went to their apartment when I got out of <u>North Shore University Hospital</u> to see the baby. I just don't remember. Yet, Lily and I will be tied together in my memory because of my pacemaker and her birth.

Privacy, Skewed Relationships and Changes

Prior to my stroke Dale never opened my mail, never looked at my bills, never looked at the <u>Empire Insurance</u> claims for Erick and me and she never looked at any contracts and money received from clients. That privacy was sacrosanct both to me and Dale.

That relationship changed from the day of my stroke until now (August 22, 2006). It was not Dale's fault. She wasn't malicious, she wasn't snooping, and she wasn't inquisitive. It was the reality of the stroke. Dale looked at my bills and claims and checks paid to me by clients. There were bills to pay and claims to look at. She helped me to write out checks. My privacy was no longer intact or sacred. On the other side of the ledger there was Dale, her privacy was respected in all ways. There was an unequal relationship. There was a double standard, a skewed twisted double standard. That was not Dale's doing. It was that nasty stroke of mine.

When I wrote this chapter I asked Dale her views on this matter. She was straightforward. She didn't want to be responsible for anyone including me. Remember this was still raw for both of us as we talked and walked the path of the past four years. She wanted me to get well as quickly as possible so that she wouldn't have to do all these tedious chores for me. Both Dale and I knew in our heart that it would be a matter of limited time before I would take more control of my life. Each day I took more control of my life each time I opened my own mail or wrote a check or looked at junk mail.

Today, August 23, 2006, I still have to ask Dale to read mail for me from <u>Nelnet</u> for the Federal Family Education Loan Program. I just want to make sure that I didn't miss anything that would cause any problems for Erick's loans. Dale also helps me when I get a voice message on my phone. I am able to get two or three numbers but not nine in one shot. I have to keep redialing and redialing until I get the numbers in place. Many times I ask Dale to write the number for me but only after I tried. Sometimes people talk fast or talk with accents. This too deals with privacy, control and power.

One of the tangential benefits of my stroke was that I spent most of my time listening to people and not talking. I listened to the wonderful banter of family and friends. I listened to the love of the loved. I listened to the actions of love, respect, and honor personified by Jeff and Anne. They listened to me and heard me and gave me the time to express my thoughts fully. They asked nothing but love, respect and honor in return.

Friends, Changes and Camouflage

The most difficult changes for me, the ones that pained me most, and the ones that made me aware that I became a different person as a result of my stroke, were the ones that altered my relationships with old friends and good acquaintances. These were the people who nurtured me in the months after my stroke but once I became more able the relationships changed. It changed because of me and it changed because of them. The changes, in retrospect, came quickly. I can't speculate or talk for others but I can tell you my thoughts.

I was not the person I was prior to my stroke and I wasn't the person I was during the early months in rehabilitation. I was a different person, a more no-nonsense, practical, focused person, not hesitating and no longer looking at all sides when a path was clear.

Maybe it was the subtleties incumbent in most of the friendships. In some we had a closeness of belief in the broad issues of the day but there were fine points that separated us. We agreed on most of the issues. Yet the nuances, as few as they were, dominated our talks. As an illustration we talked about the historical benefits about Christianity and we agreed on about ninety-nine percent of the issues that we talked about. Then we chatted about Catholicism and Protestantism and we agreed on about eighty percent of the thoughts under discussion. Then we conversed about the intricacies between Lutherans, Methodists, and Episcopalians and we were in accord less than fifty percent of the time. Finally we spoke about the minutiae between the Lutherans split into the Missouri Synod and the Evangelical Lutheran Church of America (ELCA) and we agreed on nothing other than to agree to disagree. And voila we hardly see or talk anymore.

As I got better two issues, two sides of the same coin, became paramount to me. They changed my relations with good friends and acquaintances. Prior to my stroke I was a private person. I never shared all my thoughts with anyone in earnest except a psychiatrist in the 1980's. For 64 years my brains whirled around my head and as I got older and older the rotations twirled faster and faster. After my stroke my brain slowed down. People who cared about me asked me about my health, rehabilitation and more intimate questions, my thoughts, my daily activities, and a continuum of brain stumping queries.

Once I got better, stronger, I smarted over the unequal relationships. Here were people who had a healthy concern about me and yet slowly, but surely, I wanted my privacy back. I didn't want to share my thoughts anymore. I didn't want to answer any of the queries as if I didn't have a choice. There were the kinds of questions asked to children or people with borderline intelligence with the expectations of answers. There wasn't a quid pro quo. I didn't want to know the details of their life, just give me the executive summary and that would be enough for me. I cared but I didn't relish all the details. In other words I didn't want to allow good friends, especially those concerned with me, to poke my mind and pry into my deepest thoughts. And that was what good friends did, not maliciously but innocently, sympathetically.

Initially, I was grateful to the people who helped me to speak more fluently but, after a couple of months, I was upset with them also. I wasn't able to finesse both feelings. My anger to my stroke was clear but after venting my fury it was important for me to do something to strengthen myself. I needed to get help daily and to allow people to help me in ways that I needed to be helped. I knew that I needed them because I was not able to control my life in a meaningful way. I couldn't speak, read or write for the first four months after my stroke. I didn't know what medicines I had to take for the morning and night. I reached out to these people and they responded with compassion. But I had to work hard by myself for myself. Those people were wonderful, they called me almost every morning, talked to me when I couldn't speak and they allowed me to try as hard as I could to say a couple of words. I prized the time they gave to me so that I could work on my conversational speech. It was true of the professional staff who worked with me for 15 months, my wife, Dale, Jeff, Anne, Pierre, friends and acquaintances.

My stroke took away my control of my life and power. It was the stroke not all the people who loved and cared for me. Yet, I focused on the sights, real and imaginary, of the people who gave me their energy, time and love.

These thoughts of mind were convoluted. I needed to get these straight in my brain. Once I got better I felt that I was more sensitive about frailties of others and yet more caustic when friends and acquaintances shared thoughts and comments with me. I was biting. I disagreed with their ideas. I tried to dissect their comments. It wasn't because I was adamant on thoughts or unyielding on issues. It was because I wanted to feel that I was unique again. I didn't want to see myself as a caricature, one that answered questions and never disagreed with comments because of my stroke and aphasia. Yes. No. Smile. I didn't want to feel like a dog or a drifter given a temporary home by a sympathetic person for reasons I couldn't phantom. This happened over months.

Let me share some illustrations of changes that caused me anguish. One of the turning points for me was when I was offended when I had a conversation with a friend and that friend asked me whether I knew something, a word/event. I said that I did. The friend proceeded to interrogate me about the word/event. I didn't answer the person, mainly because the word/event was commonplace and by grilling me, and it was a grilling, it demeaned both my knowledge and integrity. Our conversation was, from my point of view, a conversation by equals. I thought that he had no right to do that. I had no time for this kind of friendship or this one up-man-ship. And yet I couldn't be sure that my take on this whole situation was accurate and fixable.

At the same time some good people felt that I owed them what I didn't know. I was grateful for their empathy, the generosity for their time and their patience and a whole host of things. And I did and I said that numerous times. I felt it. I conveyed it to them. But as I got more comfortable with conversational speech there were changes. Initially, it was funny when someone deliberately spoke quickly to me so that the person could get control over our conversation. Sometimes it was used to poke fun at me, especially when there was another person listening to our discussions. Finally, it wasn't funny at all. It was down right nasty. That happened when my thoughts were lucid, focused and well presented. Some people were threatened as I made my comeback and our relationships changed.

The New Year 2003: Birth, Death, Inequities, a Minuscule Sample of Life's Cycle

By New Year 2003 I nearly finished the first year cycle of my stroke. I could speak with limitations, read slowly, and write with severe hardship. I had a good business with better prospects. I wished it was a healthy, happy, successful year for all the people I loved and their loved ones. I wished for peace also. It was a stereotypical wish of a Miss America contestant or a politician but it was also my wish.

It was at this point that Dale was stretched to her emotional and physical limits. She worked five days a week. She cared for me as much as I resented and hated that thought. It was true. She took care of me. Over the years I realized how remarkable she was to do all she did for me with kindness, refinement, composure and beauty. But it was even more incredible because she had to care for her father at the same time, sometimes at our home and in the last months of his life at a hospital after work during weekdays and in the day on the weekends. Dale's father was a good, unruffled, strong, sweet gentleman and Dale loved him immensely. I felt so distressed for Dale when he died.

Over the past year Dale shared many of her thoughts with me and her pain is so intense when she relives those days. As she shares those memories I quaked silently with grief, desolation and melancholy and I now know why she dreads reading this manuscript. It is jam-packed with the good and the pain of life but the pain is the vulnerable, the fear of lost love, the things that will never be again, memories, touches of skin, shared laughter, and thoughts. As she and I talk I learn so much about the depths of her soul, the love within her and the pain she feels because she has and gives love freely.

It was about this time that I read Stephen Hawking's <u>A Brief History of Time</u>. I thought I had a general understanding of who Hawking was but that wasn't true.

That understanding was about his illness and physical limitations and the pictures of him in magazines in his wheelchair and the gadgets that he used for communicating his vast knowledge of physics and astronomy. That was all I knew of him. I focused on his illness and unbelievable handicaps. It was the picture of the poster boy trying to achieve against overwhelming odds. I wanted to know how he was able to make the world notice him when in my world people preferred not to see faces that can't speak, read, or write, faces that are thrown away.

It took me about two-three months to read A Brief History of Time. I had to read every word in the book aloud and slowly. I remember one day, it was cold but sunny, and I went to a park in Manhasset after I finished working with Peggy for the day. I just wanted to get away from my world for a couple of hours. I took the book with me and I found a bench in the warm sun away from the few people in the park. The reason that I remembered the scene in my mind was that I was amazed and proud that I was able to pronounce nearly all the words in the pages that I read and I was able to put a couple of words together and read them fluently aloud.

I can't say that I understood the whole book, I didn't but I got a better picture of the universe. There were words that I had to relearn, "big bang", "black holes", and "wormholes" and many others that I never knew and didn't understand. I improved my vocabulary. But I was proud that I read the book. I knew that I wouldn't have read it if I didn't have my stroke.

As I read this book I knew that he was a unique scientist and person. He was acknowledged by his peers throughout the world and awarded the most prestigious prizes in his disciple. He was a fighter as tenacious as a person could be to fight his diseased body. He brought knowledge to people throughout the world about the universe. He was brilliant, courageous, and inspirational. Everything that was done to help him was important and warranted the special wheelchair, the voice box, and all the other technological gadgets that made his life better and productive. No questions about that.

And yet when I marveled at his accomplishments I wondered about myself and all of the stroke and brain trauma victims at <u>Transitions of Long Island</u> and the hundreds of thousands of other people in the country, the ones who had to fight insurance companies to get more time for their rehabilitation or get computers and other gadgets that would allow them to be more productive in their lives. They and I, we, wanted to be "whole" and our loved ones wanted us to be made "whole". Yet the government didn't fight for us and insurance companies and their lobbyists and lawyers fought against us so that their profits were higher. How many more people could improve their lives for the cost of a couple of bombs or tanks or bullets? And why don't we require insurance companies to make sure that everyone has at least the same care given to a Hawking, Gates, yes and even the Bush clan and congress?

February 17, 2003 to May 30, 2003: The Discharge

I saw Peggy once or twice a week for one hour daily from February 17 to May 30, 2003. I was prepared for my discharge from <u>Transitions of Long Island</u>. These were not academic questions for me but real life issues. I still flounder for words when I am in conversation and this is September 3, 2006 three years and four months after I "graduated" from <u>Transitions of Long Island</u>. I still am not able to read rapidly with fluency to my grandchildren and I still am not able to put the correct inflections in the stories that I read to them and this is September 3, 2006 three years and four months after I "graduated" from <u>Transitions of Long Island</u>. I still am not comfortable in situations when I have to deal with a barrage of questions and answers and this is September 3, 2006 three years and four months after I "graduated" from <u>Transitions of Long Island</u>. I still need to ask people on the phone and in person to say a telephone number one number at a time and do that slowly and this is September 3, 2006 three years and four months after I "graduated" from <u>Transitions of Long Island</u>. I still need to use my computer and its thesaurus to write letters, e-mails and this book if not word by word at least for one word in a sentence and this is September 3, 2006 three years and four months after I "graduated" from <u>Transitions of Long Island</u>. Please don't get me wrong. I made tremendous gains at <u>Transitions of Long Island</u>. I can speak, read, and write. Yet I wonder everyday if I would have made even greater gains, in a more efficient and effective manner, if I had spent more time in <u>Transitions of Long Island</u>?

In the report by Peggy Kramer and Jean Elbaum, Ph.D, <u>Progress Report and Discharge Summary Donald Weinstein,</u> May 30, 2003, they said that I had demonstrated a high degree of motivation. They noticed that I made consistent gains in receptive and expressive language. They judged my expressive language skills as "normal". I don't think that "normal" was equal to "whole" as in "made whole". With more time with Peggy could I have made more gains in a more efficient and effective manner? Were the lines drawn by the insurance company to determine when I had enough rehabilitation subjective and arbitrary and who benefited from those criteria but the insurance company? The report pointed out that I demonstrated gains in confrontational naming, verbal fluency, and verbal specificity. Does the word "gains" equal "whole" as in "made whole"? When the report "demonstrated significant gains" in my reading and writing, vocabulary, processing speed, memory, eye contact and confidence did that equate with "whole" as in "made whole"? That was good for the insurance company but not for me. The report said that I was an "effective and functional" communicator. Do the words "effective and functional" communicator equal "whole" as in "made whole"? To the insurance company it did but not to me. I had to live with its unilateral decisions and standards. I knew that I still had problems with finding words, some stuttering, and severe problems with numbers. In a re-evaluation of me, on May 1, 2003, thirty days before

I was discharged from Transitions of Long Island, I "demonstrated mild receptive language deficits, particularly in the area of auditory recall at the sentence level for details such as dates and times." The report said that "During unstructured discourse, occasional pauses are demonstrated due to residual word finding." The insurance company didn't ask me my thoughts about whether I would be better off if I spent more time at Transitions of Long Island. And finally the report said that "Dr. Weinstein is agreement with discharge at this time as he has attained all goals." The report was written by people I trusted and still trust. Peggy and I and our spouses have socialized three or four times since I graduated from Transitions of Long Island. I never asked her if I would have made more gains if I spent more time at Transitions of Long Island. Was there pressure on Transitions of Long Island to discharge me by the insurance company? Could I have realistically known and predicted 15 months after my stroke all the goals and objectives needed to make me "whole" and the time and energy needed to get closer and closer to the person I was before my stroke? I think not.

As I wrote this part of the book, September 5, 2006, it was clear to me that the insurance company never planned to help make me "whole". It used words such as "gains", "significant gains", "normal", "mild", "mildly" for a paper trail, a paper trail used by bureaucratic businesses concerned by legal suits. They never really planned to help me to achieve my goal of "wholeness". They wanted to show the courts, if necessary, that through Transitions of Long Island, I was able to get part of my speech, reading and writing skills back. They were not concerned about the maximum skills I needed to become "whole", those were more costly in time and services. They wanted to get me to a level that they judged by their standards was "normal" at the most minimal cost. They didn't allow me to get rehabilitation classes in "cognition" even though Transitions of Long Island said that I needed this service. They didn't teach me to re-read Spanish when that was a significant part of my intellectual being. The point that I have made is that insurance premiums get paid but the insurance companies are the arbitrators of what service will be provided. Don't allow that to happen to you and your loved one.

Language and Travel

Dale and I went to Puerto Rico, from February 14 to 21, 2003, for her school winter break and one of our anniversaries. Anne and Jeff gave us one of their timeshare weeks as a gift. We had a great time. The temperature was somewhere in the 80s. The complex where we stayed was lovely. It looked over a narrow channel with yachts; the early sun wrapped by a clear beautiful blue sky filled the balcony where we ate breakfast. Most of the rest of the mornings and afternoons we went to beach and took in the sun and swam in the green blue waters of the Caribbean.

There were times that we went sightseeing. We rented a car and drove over to El Yunque, the tropical forest, and enjoyed the sights of the waterfall. We rode a municipal bus to and from old San Juan. I knew that many people, especially in the shops and restaurants in San Juan and in the complex where we resided were fluent in English. At first I was reluctant to speak Spanish, I wasn't sure that I could get the words out of my mouth and I worried about my stuttering. Within a couple of minutes after we arrived at the complex we wanted to know whether the room was ready for us. The maid was not an English speaking person. I used verbs to get my thoughts across. It worked. While we drove to El Yunque we got hungry for lunch. We pulled over and went into a Subway and I ordered a ham and cheese sandwich in Spanish because the clerk indicated that he didn't speak English. It wasn't much but it was something. By the time Dale and I wanted to sightsee in San Juan I was more comfortable with approaching a woman at a bus stop. It turned out that she was from Chile, she lived in Puerto Rico for awhile, but she did understand what I said in Spanish. I was able to get information on the next bus and the stop that we needed to get off. The woman was very generous and pleasant. I wasn't proficient, not even close, but those Spanish sounds were starting to become familiar to me. Dale was a great cheerleader. She told me that people understood my Spanish even though it was limited and those kisses she gave me were incentives to work hard. I loved those kisses I still love those kisses.

A Terrible Experience with a Guard and Police Officers

This section of this book deals with only about four hours out of the 5,040 hours in the seven months covered in this chapter. It was somewhere in February March 2003. Yet it gets a disproportionate share of the ink in the chapter because I still seethed even after four years because, in my mind, I was abused by an arrogant ignorant IRS guard and two police officers. There are lessons in this story for stroke survivors, caretakers, police officers and politicians. I hope so, so that my pain has some redeeming benefits for others.

Once a month I paid my overdue taxes to the IRS in person because it was a cheap way for me to get a tutor. I talked to the clerk and asked questions and the clerk spoke to me and answered my questions. I saw one or two clerks; they were regularly at the desk. This got me away from my house in the morning or afternoon too once a month. That was my thought when I went to the IRS that day no more than that.

I went to the IRS building and did what I did in the past. I said hi, but I told the guard that I couldn't pass the metal detector arch because I had a pacemaker. I was told by the nurse, Ms.Donna Kalenderian, Electrophysiology Nurse Practitioner A.N.P., where I got my pacemaker at <u>North Shore University Hospital</u>, more than once that I should not go under the metal detector and ask the person to use the wand to search me. I did that.

The genesis for the following nightmare should be put squarely on the shoulder of this guard. He was adamant that I had to go through the metal detector even after I explained to him that I was told not to use the metal detector by the hospital. He sat in his chair and did nothing. He didn't use the wand. He did nothing. I waited for twenty minutes and then I called the acting administrator in the building. I either spoke to his secretary or to a voice message box and left a message. After ten or so minutes when the acting administrator didn't come I called the police and told them that I was not able to get in to the IRS building, a guard hindered my entry and the problem. I waited for them in the front of the building.

With this scene in place the following events occurred. I informed the acting administrator and the two police officers at once that I had a stroke and I had a pacemaker and that I was told by the nurse that I should not go under the metal detector and ask the person to use the wand to search me. I had in my wallet a Cardiac Pacemaker Patient Identification Card with my name, my telephone number, the model number of the pacemaker, the serial number and the implant date of 03/Dec/2002.

I was very frustrated by the sarcastic game played by the guard and cursed, "bastard" and "fuck", at the guard for his enjoyment of this game played at my expense. This guard was making medical and electromagnet judgments and I think that the acting administrator let him do that without verifying the facts with the North Shore University Hospital or the department or agency in Federal Plaza in Manhattan that dealt with guards.

There were multi-conversations in the lobby and I couldn't follow the thoughts, answers and questions, it become overwhelming to me. The police officers heard my arguments and tried to get the acting administrator and guard to relent. They knew that security guards in the airports used wands. They knew that the clerks "knew" me and said so. No one else was in the lobby. They could have done a hand search. The guard had looked at all the items in my pockets before this. They knew exactly where I needed to go, about 100 feet from the lobby within eye sight from the lobby door.

I couldn't understand questions and comments to me when more than one person talked and/or yelled at me. That was especially true if those people talked rapidly to me or talked to me when their mouths were not facing directly at me. All of a sudden, maybe after a half hour to an hour, one of the police officers said that he had to go somewhere or do something after work.

That police officer came at me with his hands ready to hit my chest. He didn't say anything to me about what he wanted or what he wanted me to do. His menacing look said everything. It took a second or two before his hands came to my chest. Instinctively, I tried to turn my shoulder away from his push/punch to my chest where my pacemaker was implanted. I worried that I would die. In an instant each police officer took one of my arms and started walking me to the door of the building.

It was surreal. I felt faint so I fell to the floor. I was worried for my heart. There was the guard smirking sitting on his chair looking at me. There were people leaving work and they looked at me as if I was a drunk or a homeless derelict. Either one was humiliating.

I wanted to make sure that someone other than my wife and my son knew what happened to me. My lawyer's office was nearby also so I called him. I had tried to put my affairs in place recently and he and I looked at my will. I got his secretary. She listened to me and she talked to the police officer and told me to try to relax. There was an ambulance on the way to determine my condition. I think that someone gave me water.

The ambulance was a police ambulance with an EMT person. Once he made a cursory examination, while I was on the floor, he told the police officers that I in fact had a new pacemaker. That got the attention of the police officers. I think the EMT person helped me up and walked me to the ambulance. The EMT person wanted a cursory understanding of the events not the nitty-gritty details. He took my blood pressure. He hooked me to an EKG, I wasn't sure if that was the correct name of the machine but it looked like the machine in my doctor's office. He looked over the print out and said that I was safe and sound.

When I got home I was furious and I called the police complaint office and spoke to some sergeant. I tried to explain the details to him. I told him that I had a stroke and speech problems and I would have difficultly answering questions if he spoke quickly to me. But he asked me quick hurried questions. I think he said that the officers were just escorting me out of the building and I should have complied with them. There were two thoughts that crossed my mind. This sergeant was not an honest broker. He made judgments before he spoke to me and it was clear that he spoke to the police officers or union representatives. His questions were slanted from my point of view. The pressured questions were meant to hassle me. He said that he wrote the answers that I gave him and I should come to his office or he would come to my house and I would sign the complaint. Either I asked him to read the statement that he wrote or he voluntarily offered to read the statements. Either way I took exception to his interpretations of what I said I said. I told him so. It was his mannerism on the phone and attitude. It was the fact that he pushed me in our conversation. I couldn't get all the words out of my mouth that I needed to finish my thoughts. I couldn't find the detailed words with the nuances needed to explain what happened to me. He made me upset again.

That day or the next day I spoke to my lawyer. His perceptions were sound for anyone but especially for me, a stroke victim with aphasia. He said that I had more than my share of pain and that this was not worthwhile. He reminded me that I should focus on my life not on a couple of police officers and my anger at them. The next day, after he spoke to a colleague of the sergeant, he told me that the whole issue was over.

I had a mixed reaction. I was glad that I didn't have to go through the hassles of the ups and downs of all the steps of a trial. It would take too much time and energy. If the police administrators didn't understand what their officers did than shame on them. At the same time I felt a loss. I was humiliated and derogated when all I wanted to do was to improve my speech and conversational speech in a safe environment. I wanted to make sure that I was safe. A security guard would have put my life in danger maybe and an acting administrator and a couple of police officers failed to verify the correct way to search and protect me.

But there was more than a glimmer of hope when I realized that night when I walked to my car and passed by one of the officers in his car and I chastised him for his actions that I had faith in myself. I was able to shout at a police officer and that police officer was able to acknowledge his error to me privately. I respected that. And I know that as abusive as the other officer was I knew that once he knew that he had to worry about his actions either in court or by a review of his peers I had faith in the system. But most of all I was able to clean the grime off me and stand tall when I walked away from the people who caused me pain and that meant that I was able to salvage my dignity; after all I protected myself by myself by my using my brain and my faith in the system and that most police officers are good people.

Speaking, Reading and Writing

I couldn't have written a letter to the police complaint board or a politician or a newspaper, in the winter of February 2003. It would have required more energy than I could have mustered. I didn't have the vocabulary at my fingers. I didn't have the idioms needed to hit the nail on the head. I couldn't have figured out the words that I needed. I couldn't have approximated the words so that the thesaurus would help me find the accurate words.

It was at this time that I read more of The Collected Stories of Isaac Babel. Babel was in the league with Kafka and the greatest Russian writers. As I read the book aloud I realized how much better a social studies teacher and college history professor I would have been if I had made my students read this book and by extension other classics that showed the events of historical eras through literary geniuses.

As always I read for vocabulary and structure. It was still a problem some times for me to read aloud and I had to reread prepositions and conjunctions over and over again to complete sentences. I was not even close to my pre-stroke vocabulary. Who could have thought that Julius Fishner's grandchild needed to relearn words that were part of my essence from the time I started talking, Shtetl, Cossacks and Talmudic? At the same time I read for content the way Babel phrased phrases and sentences.

When I read this book it took me to a world that my grandparents wanted to get away from for themselves, their children, and their grandchildren. To me Babel's stories showed the reality of the fratricide wars between red and white armies during the period of the Russian Revolution and in the "Red Cavalry Stories" that spanned the 1920s. There was more than the ugliness of the honor of war. It was the path of plain people in places where they didn't want to be with people they didn't like, appreciate or want. They were forced, uprooted, by arrogant petty men with allegiances to ideologies, the religion of state and or class. There were insignificant men and boys, women and girls, tiny unknown villages with unknown people with feelings and dreams and bigotry, rooted in religion, fear and uncertainty, all smelling the stench of war, death, and indescribably sadness. Yet there was small ray of hope for a better life.

Somewhere in my brain my wires crossed. My eyes cried for what I don't know with a visceral reaction to what I didn't know because I didn't know. I probably juxtaposed the nothingness of war and death and destitute with people like me, stroke victims, unable to do or be. I would be part of the list of people in Michael Harrington's The Other America, faceless, erased, and forgotten. This raw feeling changed insistently to white hot resentment. This country, through Universal Medical Care, could and should help stroke victims from Plymouth Rock, Massachusetts, Edmonton, New York, Zachary, Louisiana, Prescott, Arizona, Wichita, Kansas, Boise, Iowa and Anaheim, California for a fraction of the costs of bombs and bullets.

Babel's stories revealed a different Jew, not shtetl Jews in Russia but those freed by the repercussions of the revolution. I never thought that I would use Jews in the same sentences with Cossacks except when there were pogroms. But Babel wrote about free new Jewish fighters, even Jewish Cossack commanders and colorful Jewish gangsters later in "The Odessa Stories". My brain held secrets from me.

As I read I remember my mind did a lot of free associating. My mind flashed to my four uncles, three of whom I had not seen for nearly thirty years and the other one I saw maybe once every ten years. One of them was a hustler, a low class robber a thief. Another one was a gangster, a goon a bone cracker. They grew up on Amboy Street in Brownsville in Brooklyn. They never took any guff. Anyway this book made me remember my uncles, their names. I couldn't remember two of their wives and four of their children my cousins.

Now, September 23, 2006, I am able to read and comprehend most, if not all, history and literary non fictional works. I read silently most of the time especially at the beach when Dale wants to read or sleep and the sun shines brightly. There are instances when I have to read aloud a word that I can't pronounce in my head. I still need to practice reading aloud to my granddaughters and grandson. I'm able to read well aloud but not perfectly. I have to work on my rhythm, pace, variation, tone and mood so that I could be a good reader to them. That is my next task.

Conclusion

This is the concluding chapter of this book but there is no end really. As long as I can feel growth in my brain, and I do regularly, I get up in the morning and look forward to the day and that was true when I graduated from <u>Transitions of Long Island</u>. At that time, May 30, 2003, I didn't know whether I would grow and get back my life. I haven't. My life is good but there is still a battle. There is a struggle between my dignity, self-respect and my brain and ridiculous and absurd people and agencies. There is a clash in my brain about my beliefs.

I know that I made tremendous gains some of them against all odds. It was and is fantastic to know that I was and am loved in ways that I couldn't phantom before my stroke. Jeff and I got closer and closer and my love for him goes to my core. My love for Anne, Alison and Jessica knows no boundaries. Every day I think about Alison and Jessica and the fact that at one time I couldn't remember their names. I am glad to hear, every and anytime I can, about their accomplishments in school, soccer, drawing, dancing, playing the piano, play dates, pajama parties, resting, bike riding, coloring, playing dominos and reading.

Dale and I have five granddaughters and one grandson. Each and everyone allow me to kiss them on their heads when we meet, when I have the urge to squeeze them. I never imagined that marriage had so many facets, so many components, before my stroke and I never knew how much love I got and get from Dale and how much tenderness, passion and devotion I have for her. My nephew, Richard, and I got closer together and I think about his daughter Eli. She is younger than Alison but older than Jessica. She and I have good conversations on the phone. He is a first-rate person, perceptive and discerning.

Since I graduated from <u>Transitions of Long Island</u> I read <u>The Idiot</u> in a 570 page unabridged version published by Barnes & Noble. It took me about six months to finish it in 2005-6. I read it aloud word by word. Once in awhile I read a couple of words together silently but those were in the last couple of chapters. I relished reading the book every

page and every footnote. I felt pleased and sad at the same time when I finished the last word of the last page.

Most of the time, somewhere in my day, I take a breath. I am not praying. I am not a religious man. I think about the fact that I can read, write and speak. I am not "whole" but I am able to go about my business, most of the time. Everything takes more time, patience, and discipline but I get to my goals.

It was and is important for me to have my goals. My dignity and daily goals go together. Those daily goals allowed me to read The Idiot and write this book and the catharsis that came from finishing this book. I know who I am and what I am again. One of my goals is to remember that I am fortunate to be loved by so many and to give love to them often and in tangible ways. At my age and health it is wonderful to be.

Checklists

Survivor needs to:

1. Make sure that you develop a list of problems that you still have before you graduate from therapy. Ask your therapist, a month before you graduate, if he could help you if the insurance company paid. If the insurance company didn't pay would you be able to "fix" yourself by yourself? If not, could that therapist suggest a way for you to get help?

2. Be savvy when approaching or being approached by a police officer. You want to make sure that the police officer is told by you or your companion that you had a stroke and aphasia. It would be important for Police Departments to in-service their police officers about the characteristics of stroke and pacemaker survivors and the proper way to treat them. Never ever allow a rent-a-cop or security guard to set himself up as any authority period much less as a maven on pacemakers and electrophysiology.

3. Stimulate your mind and body every day. Read read read daily. Write write write daily. Speak speak speak daily. My experience is that I was able to feel my brain grow. My brain grew after I graduated from <u>Transitions of Long Island</u>. I still feel those feeling today three years and four months after I parted from <u>Transitions of Long Island</u>.

4. Make sure that you work hard to keep your dignity intact. Always prize yourself respect and essence.

Spouse and Friends need to:

1. Help your stroke survivor make a list of problems that he still has before he graduate from therapy.

2. Engage your stroke survivor in stimulating conversations and activities.

3. Enhance your stroke survivor's dignity.